Prevent Acid Reflux

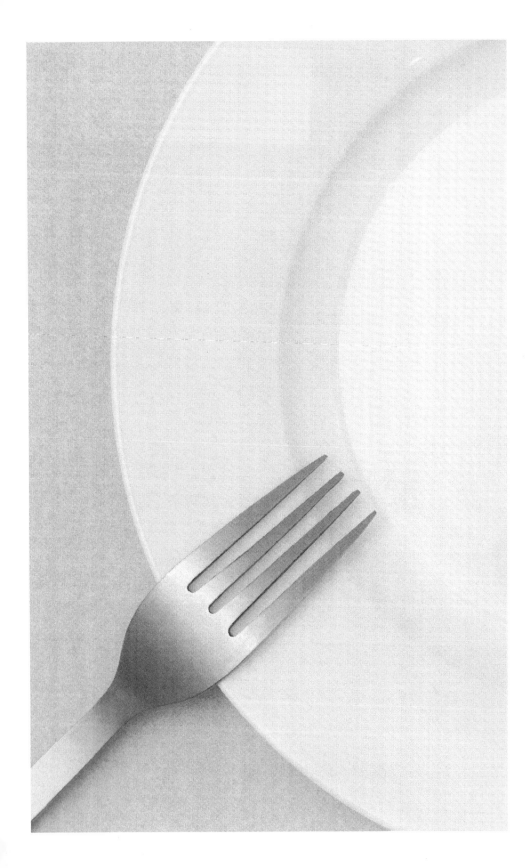

Prevent Acid Reflux

Delicious Recipes to Cure Acid Reflux and GERD

HEALDSBURG
PRESS

Contents

CHAPTER SEVEN

Soups, Salads, and Sandwiches   71

CHAPTER EIGHT

Appetizers and Side Dishes   95

CHAPTER NINE

Main Courses   109

CHAPTER TEN

Desserts   131

Introduction

The feeling is intensely unpleasant and, once felt, unforgettable. The chest burns and a bitter fluid floods the back of the throat. The taste lingers. You feel nauseous; your belly swells after a meal. Is it stomach flu? Or is it something far worse? These burning, nauseating symptoms are also part of a heart attack, you've heard. Your anxiety rises as your symptoms grow worse.

Relax. Take a deep breath. Chances are you are not having a coronary, nor are you about to take to your bed with the latest strain of influenza. Very likely you are one of millions and millions of Americans who experience acid reflux. No part of the population is safe from this disease, and by no means is it found only in older adults: pregnant women and infants often suffer too. In fact, because of obesity worldwide and the aging population of baby boomers, a 2004 study reported a 46 percent increase in acid reflux–related visits. In fact, this condition is so widespread, clinics are popping up to treat swallowing and voice disorders, all symptoms of reflux. Not surprisingly, the surge of digestive tract disorders overall is linked to the rising percentage of the population in the United States that suffers from being overweight and obese.

"Acid reflux" is the medical term given to persistent heartburn experienced more than twice a week. These "acid attacks" leave you weary and fragile with pain ranging from a mere annoyance to an insufferable burn behind the breastbone. Your throat hurts and you are coughing because the acid has escaped into your lungs. You are miserable. Unchecked, persistent heartburn becomes something quite different and dangerous: cancer of the esophagus. GERD—or gastroesophageal reflux disease—is the name given to the set of symptoms caused by ongoing acid in the tube between stomach and throat and is far more serious than occasional bouts of acid reflux. Some use the name interchangeably, but GERD develops when acid reflux becomes a chronic condition. With the help of this book, you can stop acid reflux long before it damages your health permanently.

For those who suffer occasionally, this book will offer simple lifestyle changes to eradicate the problem. For those who suffer greatly, the book will present a battle plan for a combination of lifestyle changes and medication that will improve the quality of life of the acid-reflux sufferer forever. This debilitating, painful condition can be eradicated, simply and quickly.

In this short, fact-filled look at acid reflux, we'll provide all the information you'll need to combat acid in your food pipe and bring it to a stop before it turns into something far worse. You'll learn what Western medicine can offer in the form of medication and surgery, as well as simple lifestyle changes and homeopathic treatments that soothe and heal.

Because acid reflux is triggered by overeating or eating too quickly, lack of sleep, stress, and medications, food will play a essential part in your recovery. We'll steer you toward foods that will help you feel better, foods that soothe and break down acid rather than trigger its flow. We'll explore non-acidic ingredients and how to use them to feed your family and keep them in good health. Arguments break out all the time over what the GERD mechanism is and how it works. Some say it's soft drinks that set it off, some say it's not. Still others say spiced foods trigger reflux, while other refute it. Keep both eyes open when reading news on the subject and the results of studies—the best person to talk to about anything you might read or hear is always your doctor.

Hopefully within days or weeks you'll feel your body changing. As nausea retreats there is no bitter bile, only the lingering satisfaction of a good meal. Your sleep will improve, your energy will increase, and your strength will return.

It's time to sit back down at the table and rejoin the conversation with family and friends, because food is not the enemy. If you make the right choices, food modulates the acid level in your stomach, which changes the acid level in the entire body, making your stomach and body more alkaline (able to neutralize acid) and free of the pain of acid reflux.

PART ONE

Acid Reflux Basics

CHAPTER ONE

The Medical Science Behind Acid Reflux

Medical science defines acid reflux as heartburn that occurs more than twice a week. A muscular valve known as the lower esophageal sphincter (LES) is the culprit. The LES opens to allow food into the stomach or for stomach air to escape through the mouth (sometimes called a burp).

If the LES opens too often or can no longer close tightly, acid seeps— or rises—forcing it into the esophagus (the tube that connects throat to stomach), where it chemically burns the upper abdomen and throat.

What causes acid reflux? Medical researchers define it as a condition triggered by excess: you simply have too much food in your stomach after a large meal or, in the case of pregnant women, the chronically constipated, and the obese, too much pressure applied to the stomach. This pressure causes the stomach to produce additional gastric acid that erodes the LES, allowing more and more escape (or flux) of destructive digestive fluids. In this manner, a vicious cycle is born.

Acid reflux can also be caused by medications. Some medicines prescribed by doctors loosen the esophageal sphincter just as pressure on the stomach does. If you are taking medication for asthma (theophylline or albuterol); blood pressure; heart medications such as calcium channel blockers; different forms of nitroglycerine; muscle relaxants; anti-anxiety medication; medicines for overactive bladder, diarrhea, or migraines; as well as any medication—either over the counter or from the doctor—that dries up the mouth and inhibits saliva production, you may be subject to acid reflux. Saliva breaks up stomach acid, making that common "cotton mouth" feeling a bit more dangerous than it seems.

Why is stomach acid so destructive to other parts of the digestive system? Chemically, gastric acid is made of hydrochloric acid (HCl)—historically referred to by the mysterious name of "muriate of potash"—plus potassium chloride (KCl) and sodium chloride (NaCl). The first component (HCl) is a corrosive, strong mineral acid. The next two chemical compounds (NaCl and HCl) are salt-based, and excessive intake of these has been tied to heart disease, diabetes, and gastric cancer. So the next time you salt your food, remember that you are simply compounding this already existing salt level.

This acid and two salts do not affect the cells in the stomach, because the cells were built to live in such an environment. The cells in your food pipe or esophagus, on the other hand, were not. Therein lies the inflamed, uncomfortable rub: stomach acid must remain in its own neighborhood or it pollutes the entire city.

To truly understand what causes the trauma of stomach acid hitting other parts of the body, look at pH numbers. In chemistry, "pH" is a term that describes the acidity or alkaline level—also known as the "basic" level—in aqueous solutions, whose basic component is water (and that means you, human). The pH of stomach acid registers as 1 or 2, while the pH of a healthy person is between 7.35 and 7.45, and pure water comes in at 7. That 5-to-6-point spread is behind acid reflux.

The entire planet experiences acid attacks in the phenomena called acid rain. Like a macrocosm of the human body, too much acid in air and water corrodes fauna and flora on a cellular level, choking off life. Again, the pH of pure water is 7, and in parts of ecologically challenged China and Russia, fog and rain water have registered a pH as low as 2.4. That's a very acidic level that eats away at living organisms, just as acid in your stomach travels upward and attacks healthy esophageal cells.

Researchers estimate that 20 percent of America suffers from acid reflux, with pregnant women especially vulnerable. In children, it's often experienced by infants, although it usually disappears between the ages of twelve and twenty-four months. In adults, researchers report that 5.4 out of 100 Americans suffer problems with gastric acid regularly.

Ten Signs You Might Have Acid Reflux

Acid reflux's symptoms range from the rare bout of uncontrollable hiccups to the most common symptom, an unpleasant burning in the throat and stomach. Let's go through the symptoms, and if you experience any combination with frequency, see your doctor immediately.

1. **Chest pain:** Stomach acid splashes through the LES into the food pipe and causes a burning pain in the chest that many mistake for a heart attack.

2. **Regurgitation:** A sour, bitter-tasting acid backs up in the throat or mouth.

3. **Choking sensation:** Stomach acid can rise so high it creates a feeling of choking. Acid-reflux sufferers can a suffer an attack while sleeping, which causes them to awake gasping for air.

4. **Hoarseness:** Many people believe they are getting a cold or flu but in reality, the acid from the stomach is breaching the LES, seeping into the esophagus and vocal chords. This phenomenon is called acid laryngitis.

5. **Sore throat:** Like the symptom above, sore throats are often assumed to be an allergy or cold. However, if the only symptom you have is a sore throat, odds are it's not an allergy or flu. Rather, your throat is sore from contact with stomach acid.

6. **Cough:** Like the previous two symptoms, coughing is associated with colds and allergy, but it can be triggered by acid escaping into the lungs.

7. **Trouble swallowing:** Over time, acid in the throat causes scarring, a by-product of the continuous damage and healing of the tissue in the esophagus.

8. **Dyspepsia:** Approximately one half of all acid-reflux patients experience the cluster of symptoms referred to as dyspepsia. Dyspepsia can be recognized as pain in the upper abdomen, an unpleasant fullness in the stomach, and nausea after eating.

9. **Over-salivating:** The mouth produces saliva that neutralizes stomach acid. Should acid rise, the mouth may begin secreting a good deal of saliva, anticipating an attack from the stomach.

10. **Bitter taste:** Acid rises and creates a bitter taste in the mouth that lingers.

When seeking a diagnosis for your group of symptoms, be advised that a growing number of people do not respond well to anti-reflux drugs and continue to have GERD symptoms. Gastrointestinal disorder experts believe that between 50 and 70 percent of GERD sufferers actually have NERD, or non-erosive reflux disease. NERD usually attacks younger, thinner females, and clinicians believe that in this situation, the liquid flooding the throat is actually bile from the liver.

In small children the symptoms vary slightly, and many children experience these symptoms without having acid reflux. Check with your pediatrician if you notice a failure to thrive in your child, a chronic cough, frequent infections, wheezing, sleep apnea (gasping for air while asleep), and severe vomiting, particularly green vomit, which is described by the word "bilious."

Common Medical Tests to Diagnose Acid Reflux and GERD

The most important information you can give your physician is a detailed list of your symptoms. Be aware of how frequently your attacks occur and what symptoms usually accompany each attack. Write it all down if necessary and hand it to your doctor. It's essential that you communicate; your doctor may be able to judge the situation from your description and prescribe the drugs that are best for you.

Your doctor may also want to order tests to access your situation. Familiarize yourself with the tests below and be prepared to discuss them with your physician:

Barium Swallow: This is an X-ray test that will require you to drink barium. The barium outlines your esophagus and will show the doctor where the damage lies. (Barium is a dry, chalky-white metallic powder. Water is added to it to create a thick milk shake–type drink. Once you drink it, the X-ray picks up the barium as white lines in the upper gastrointestinal tract, showing any disturbance in the physical structure of the esophagus.)

Cardiac Evaluation: If you have chest pain as one of your symptoms, your doctor may want to give you an EKG test to evaluate and treat any stress or disease of the heart.

Esophageal Manometry or Motility Study: These are tests that check for the squeezing motion of the esophagus while swallowing.

Esophageal pH Monitoring: This test uses electrodes to measure the acid levels (pH) in the esophagus, usually over a twenty-four-hour period. As described in chapter 3, acid reflux requires more alkaline (less acidic) food and drink that will ensure the environment in the upper gastrointestinal tract is combating acid flux effectively.

At-Home Test for GERD

A great home tool for controlling acid in the system is the pH strip. You can test your saliva or urine with a pH strip, monitoring your pH levels from day to day. If you register below 5.6, start the Acid Reflux Diet as soon as possible—tomorrow morning, if you can. Good drugstores, health food markets, and general retailers such as Wal-Mart carry the strips, and you can order from large online retailers sites such as www.amazon.com and www.drugstore.com. In most cases, the strips cost between ten and fifteen dollars. Depending on the outcome of conversations with your physician and your medical tests, you can make a determination together about a treatment strategy. Then with this book you'll have an eating plan to supplement your medical intervention, a powerful two-fisted punch to keep acid down in the stomach where it belongs.

Common Treatments and Medications Your Doctor May Prescribe

When you discuss your symptoms with your doctor, he or she may offer three tools in the battle against escaped acid. Depending on the stage and severity of your reflux, you will be presented with behavior modification (lifestyle changes), medication, and surgery. Let's take a look at the medication first.

Your doctor will prescribe one of three medication types to treat acid reflux based on the frequency and intensity of your symptoms. They are antacids, H-2 receptor blockers, and proton pump inhibitors.

Antacids are usually prescribed for the occasional bout of acid reflux. This drug neutralizes acidity and inhibits the activity of pepsin, an enzyme produced in the stomach that is active only in an acidic environment. Two of the fastest-acting antacids are sodium bicarbonate (baking soda) and magnesium hydroxide (milk of magnesia). Unfortunately, these two fast-acting drugs have the shortest lifespan of all the antacids.

The two antacids that act more slowly but last longer are aluminum hydroxide (Alternagel, Alu-Cap, Alu-Tab, and Amphojel) and calcium carbonate (Alka-Mints, Caltrate 600, Rolaids, Tums, and Calcid). Check the label for details and choose which type of antacid is best to control your symptoms.

H-2 receptor blockers work differently than antacids by reducing the production of acid in the stomach, thus reducing the overall acidity and allowing the esophagus to heal. There are four types of H-2 receptor blockers commonly prescribed for acid reflux: cimetidine (Tagamet HB), famotidine (Pepcid AC), ranitidine (Zantac), and nizatidine (Axid). These drugs are usually prescribed for a period of eight to twelve weeks. The H-2 receptor drugs have been tested extensively, have been proven incredibly safe, and can be taken for longer periods of time to heal deep, chronic gastric acid and its more serious companion, GERD.

The third type of prescription acid-reflux medication is the proton pump inhibitor, or PPI. The strongest of all gastric acid–reducing medications, PPIs inhibit the protein pump in the gastric parietal cells, suppressing the acid-mediated breakdown of proteins in the stomach. These powerful medications can make the user more susceptible to bone fractures over time and can elevate the risk of food allergies due to undigested proteins. Common generics prescribed in the PPI class of drugs are omeprazole (Prilosec, LOMAC, and Gasec) and lansoprazole (Prevacid, Zoton, and Levant). Also keep watch for imidazopyridine derivatives, the latest drug currently undergoing promising new research in the protein pump inhibitors class of drugs.

Surgery is required when acid reflux continues to burn the esophagus, even with the use of medication. The incessant reflux creates scars that cause a narrowing of the esophagus, making it difficult to eat, so laser surgery is used to open up the food pipe.

The most commonly performed procedure for GERD is called fundoplication surgery. It takes the upper curve of the stomach (the fundus) and wraps it around a portion of the esophagus. Then the stomach and esophagus are sewn in place, creating a barrier to the acid. Endoscopic surgery binds the esophagus to the top of the stomach with stitches, staunching the flow of acid. Radiofrequency treatments are sometimes used as well. This procedure calls for waves of energy hitting the esophagus wall, which creates small amounts of scarring. This physician-created and calibrated scar tissue reduces acid reflux symptoms.

In the case of strictures—scarring of the esophagus that blocks the smooth digestion of food—doctors will treat any underlying infection with antibiotics before undertaking surgery. Once the infection clears, a surgeon inserts a bougie, a weighted tube that reopens the esophagus.

A promising new surgical procedure is to implant a LINX device, an expandable ring of metal beads that keeps stomach acid from refluxing into the esophagus. This device is one of the newest weapons in the war on acid reflux, and the Mayo Clinic in Florida is the first to offer the implant. (At the moment, certain insurance companies still classify the LINX system as an experimental protocol.)

Most surgical procedures for GERD are extremely safe. However, certain dangers increase any time you open the human body, especially in the germ-rich environment of a hospital. If medication fails, move on to surgery as a last resort.

All surgery considerably increases the chance of infection and/or mortality. The incidence of site infections after surgery is unknown because only twenty-one states in America are required to make that information public. By best estimates, 100,000 people die from hospital-induced infections each year. General anesthesia kills seven in one million patients during the procedure. In the year following the application of anesthesia, the mortality rate rises sharply: one in twenty will die within the first year, and among those aged sixty-five and over, the rate rises to one in ten.

The Health Risks of Sustained Acid Reflux and Continued Use of Antacids

Sustained acid reflux becomes GERD, a larger, more profound set of symptoms, which can then turn to esophagitis, a permanent damaging of the lining of the esophagus. This then turns into Barrett's esophagus, the precursor to throat or esophageal cancer (cells are beginning to change at this final stage before cancer). Finally, if the continuous acid exposure damages and changes cells in the food pipe, you'll be fighting esophageal and throat cancer. Only 10 percent of acid-reflux sufferers develop Barrett's esophagus, but 10 percent is high enough. In short, continued digestive trauma dominates—and ruins— other healthy systems in the body as well as day-to-day life.

Though not completely understood, acid reflux left unchecked can trigger the onset of many respiratory problems, including asthma, chronic bronchitis, chronic sinusitis, emphysema, and pulmonary fibrosis. Acid reflux also destroys tooth enamel.

Most drugs have side effects, as most of America has learned from television commercials, where pharmaceutical companies are required to list potential—and usually horrifying—health problems triggered by the drug. Speak with your doctor, as he or she needs to take your entire health profile under consideration when prescribing your medication.

Over-the-counter medications can create as many challenges as some prescribed drugs. If you are self-medicating for long periods of time with over-the-counter antacids, you should see a doctor, as you may need a stronger, more effective medication or perhaps even surgery.

Taking over-the-counter antacids for long periods of time puts your health at risk. First, antacids can cause adverse reactions when combined with other drugs (tetracycline, amphetamines, and the antifungal ketoconazole are a few), which can further damage health.

Second, prolonged antacid use can damage the stomach over time, destroying important stomach bacteria that fight off infection. To maintain good health, your stomach possesses a particular ecology, including bacteria that help break down food and keep the entire digestive system flowing. Kill certain bacteria with long-term antacid usage and you will disrupt the flow. A disrupted flow in turn leads to scarring and blockage and a resurgence of acid-reflux symptoms.

Over-the-counter antacids are simply not intended for long-term use. Rather, they are for infrequent bouts of heartburn, and will simply cloak symptoms that indicate the problem is growing worse.

Ten Simple Steps to Reduce Acid-Reflux Symptoms

After discussing your course of medication with your doctor, you can make simple lifestyle changes that will decrease the acid in your esophagus and promote its healing. Used alongside medication and diet, these changes should help substantially reduce, if not heal, your acid reflux. Here are ten ideas to put to work in your life right now:

1. **Do not go to bed with a full stomach.** The Spanish eat dinner at 10 p.m., but you shouldn't—not if you're going to bed immediately after. Allow yourself several hours after a meal to digest it and decrease the amount of food in your stomach. A full stomach in an inert human will exert pressure on the LES, compromising its function. The acid will rise and you may flux, startling you out of sleep with a choking sensation.

2. **Limit fluids at meals.** Fluid adds volume to whatever is in your stomach, so the more you drink, the more the food in your stomach swells. A swollen stomach exerts pressure on the food tube, forcing acidic bile up and through the LES. Limit your intake at meals. Take a walk. Let your food begin its process through the body before drinking large amounts.

3. **Eat less, slowly.** When it comes to eating, slow down. Taking smaller bites, chewing your food, and leaving time between mouthfuls all help to keep your stomach from becoming too full, exerting pressure up through the food pipe, and triggering reflux. In addition, try to decrease your portion sizes. If you are still hungry, get more food. But you need to learn to register your fullness and stop eating. Another strategy is especially helpful when eating out: eat half or two-thirds of what's on your plate, then stop and ask yourself if you are full. If the answer is yes, have the waitstaff remove the food in front of you. "Out of sight, out of mind," as they say.

4. **Cut the fat.** Fatty foods and grease relax the LES. When the LES relaxes, liquid gets through. That liquid is stomach acid that causes heartburn. Deep-fried foods and fatty cuts of meat such as pastrami, bacon, and pork belly should all be struck from your personal menu. When you recover, these should be only occasional treats.

5. **Do not lie down for two hours following a meal.** Just as you shouldn't go to sleep right after a meal, lying down encourages stomach acids to flow in the wrong direction. Remember, gravity is your friend. Avoid the couch and sit up for a couple hours, helping your food flow downward into the stomach where, hopefully, it stays.

6. **Chew cinnamon or fruit-flavored gum after meals.** Saliva neutralizes stomach acid, and chewing gum stimulates the production of saliva. However, take note: Do not chew mint gum. Mint is a trigger food for acid reflux, while cinnamon slows digestion, which in turn keeps a rush of food from pressing against the LES and triggering reflux.

7. **Lose weight.** While easier said than done, even a tiny bit of weight loss will help relieve pressure on the LES. By controlling portions and how fast you eat, some natural weight loss should occur. Your clothes become looser—especially at the waist—and this helps keep the pressure off the stomach as well. Clothes that are tight at the waist only add more pressure to the stomach, intensifying your symptoms.

8. **Move.** It's essential to get your body moving, especially after eating. Vigorous exercise such as running will irritate the digestive tract, so walk. Moderate, low-impact exercise will keep the digestive tract moving, a fact known to those who take an after-dinner walk regularly. Work in up to thirty minutes of walking a day, and you'll notice improved digestion.

9. **Avoid trigger foods.** In chapters 2 and 3, you'll learn a lot about foods that trigger acid reflux and how to eat to heal. Foods you should avoid include caffeine, mints of any kind, tomatoes, spicy foods, onions, garlic, carbonated beverages, and, sadly, chocolate.

10. **Quit smoking.** Smoking limits saliva production, the body's natural defense against stomach acid. Actually, any activity that dries out your mouth and inhibits the production of saliva will contribute to acid reflux pain and damage.

As you can see, the acid-reflux sufferer has many options for recovery. As the body rebuilds, the LES tightens, and symptoms recede, you will be able to resume eating some of your favorite foods occasionally and in moderation. Make your doctor your partner in fighting acid reflux. With a combination of effective drugs, modified diet, and a few changes to your lifestyle, you can put this condition behind you. You will feel strong, healthy, and symptom-free, and meals will again be a pleasure instead of a catalyst for intense, burning pain.

CHAPTER TWO

Acid Reflux and Diet

As we discussed before, GERD is a disease of excess. You are eating too much food—often foods that trigger your disease—and too much food causes pressure on the stomach. That pressure opens up your LES. Acid escapes through the LES and wrecks the esophagus, throat, and mouth because the cells aren't immune to the effects of stomach acid. Discomfort and pain are your constant companions.

GERD is also triggered by stress, an ever-present reality of twenty-first-century life. You will need to learn to slow down around mealtimes, leave more time between bites, and move your body after eating. You may need to adjust your thinking about what creates a meal and how many times a day you should eat. You will have to make time to process your food more slowly and save your health.

The tremendous news is that food can literally change your DNA. By making specific food choices, you turn your health on and off, helping or harming life at the cellular level. The right foods help cells discharge toxins, keeping them intact and healthy. Make poor choices, and toxins build in the cells, causing them to change. These cells, mutated by toxins, will eventually turn to cancer.

Since you have to eat to stay alive, GERD sufferers who make adjustments in what they eat and how they eat are the most successful at overcoming this disease. As the saying goes, "Know thyself," for not only are there common food triggers, but also each person has different chemistry, along with foods that may cause the esophagus to flux. Awareness of foods that make you sick is key.

As in many weight-loss programs, experts suggest you keep a "food log" of what you have consumed. It's a good idea if you have acid reflux as well. Just take a piece of paper, write "no" in big letters across the top, and make a list of every food that creates an acid surge in your system. Don't eat those foods—even if they are your favorites—until your symptoms subside. Then, limit yourself to eating them occasionally and in great moderation. After all, there is simply no point in eating something that makes you sick, no matter how delicious it tastes. Any momentary pleasure is lost in a storm of acid-reflux pain.

Many diets suggest you chew your food slowly and carefully. The reason for this is twofold. First, if you chew slowly, you avoid sending a huge load of food into the stomach, triggering a surge of acid. By sending the food down more slowly, the stomach produces a smaller amount of acid, which means it is less likely to back up into your food pipe. If you chew slowly, your stomach will keep pace with your mouth, and food will not back up in your system.

Second, if you chew more slowly, you will truly taste your food, and you'll feel more satisfied and alive. Simply put, the human body was not built to jam a hamburger into the pipeline before leaving the drive-through line. Your body needs time to digest food and turn it into energy: in short, make time for your food, or you will continue to suffer. In addition to recognizing your list of trigger foods, be aware of the conditions under which you eat. If you are too rushed, find a quieter spot to eat at a more leisurely pace. Do not eat meals in the car or while you focus on a computer screen, a phone call, or contentious co-workers. In other words, be kind to yourself—you deserve a little time. Unconscious eating (shoving food into your mouth when you are not hungry or even aware) is a significant element of this disease.

While it sounds strange, most people are not conscious of what they eat every day. That's fine if they do not suffer reflux, but you—at least until you get your symptoms under control—will not heal if you keep exposing your system to the irritating foods that produce acid flux. Just as you would remove grit digging into your eye, you need to remove what fills the back of your mouth with bitterness and burning.

You will have a great deal of power over your recovery if you simply make a few easy adjustments in your approach to eating. Here are a few ideas that might help:

- **Keep your own "trigger foods list" and carry it with you.** It's easy to forget that a radish caused heartburn two weeks ago. If you have the list with you, you can double-check for offending foods and add to it as you go.

- **Make portion sizes smaller**, allowing your stomach to process food at its own pace. If you swallow a large amount of food in a small amount of time, the digestive system backs up, forcing acid up the pipe.

- **Try eating smaller meals with more frequency.** No one, except possibly your mother or the armed forces, demands that you eat three meals a day. Try breaking your three daily meals into four or five smaller ones. You'll consume the same amount of food over a longer period of time, giving the stomach plenty of time to work. This will decrease backup and blockage that forces the LES open, allowing acid to flux into your upper abdomen, throat, and mouth.

- **Find a restful space to eat and enjoy your food.** This is easier said than done. If you have a demanding job or are raising kids, slowing down long enough to eat might be a seemingly insurmountable challenge. Be flexible. If you notice the first time your day slows down is 2 p.m., eat then when you have the time. If there is no break, experiment with tiny meals taken more frequently. Step out of the action and try to get away from electronic beeping, blinking lights, and demanding people. Allow yourself to eat calmly, chewing every bite. Multitasking and eating are like texting and driving for the GERD sufferer: they just don't mix.

- **Enlist helpers.** If you are in charge of food in your house, you can make dietary changes easily. If you're not, sit down with the cook. Photocopy your list of trigger foods and explain your problem. People love to be needed and will usually help. At work, confide in a co-worker for support and, when someone teases you for not having your regular four donuts at the meeting, you'll have someone to wink at across the conference table. Don't be bullied into "just one enchilada" if it means you will suffer.

- **Learn to feel good.** Focus on how you react to foods, and put aside anything that triggers your symptoms. Don't settle for feeling good occasionally. If you give yourself enough time to heal, you will be completely pain-free and perhaps even able to eat foods on your trigger list occasionally.

How the Acid Reflux Diet Works

Eating to tame acid reflux and GERD is not a diet per se: it's a strategy to promote healing and health. There is no measuring or weighing of food, nor is there a sense of denying yourself. Quite simply, if you eat whole foods that have been cooked without large quantities of fat, you will thrive. Persist in eating deep-fried or processed foods, on the other hand, and you will continue to suffer.

By combining medication and eating modification, you will heal. Once you've begun to heal, you can start reintroducing your favorite foods *in moderation*. So relax—in your future, there just may be an onion ring with your name on it.

Here are the primary strategies for the Acid Reflux Diet:

1. **Avoid bad fats.** In a strange twist of literal thinking, someone declared "fat makes you fat" years ago, and weight-conscious people everywhere began to cut all fats from their diet. Now science has told us that there are good fats and bad fats. Good fats promote your body's functions, and bad fats—like a vat of hot, melted lard crisping up your fries—inhibit or halt essential functions. An avocado, on the other hand, is full of good fat that keeps the machine—your body—greased and humming.

2. **Eat real food.** Lettuce is real food; a deep-fried fruit pie is not. Seems simplistic? Not at all. Processed foods inform every part of life. And what makes a food "processed"? For our purposes here, "processed" equals "bad fats and chemicals." Read the label. All the ingredients listed should be something you can buy, not chemical additives such as guar gum, BHT, and BHA—chemicals that preserve fats in the marketplace. Remember: The food industry is focused on money, not your health. They want their products to remain for sale for as long as possible on the supermarket shelf, so stop giving them your money to make you sick. The only one who is going to make the right food choices for you is you.

3. **Give your taste buds time to love whole foods.** Your love of fast and processed foods is not your fault. The food industry has made it their job to get you hooked. How do they do it? By constantly fiddling with levels of fat, salt, and sugar, which creates an addiction-like environment—it's wired to make you want more and more. If you wean yourself from extra bad fats, sugar, and salt, your satisfaction level adjusts to these new tastes and reacts accordingly. Once everything you eat is real, you'll discover different textures, colors, and tastes. Real food will also flood your body with the nutrients it needs to perform. Feeling good may feel funny at first, but keep going. Soon real food will be all you crave, and a sip of a diet Coke will taste like something you buy at a gas station.

4. **Avoid trigger foods.** Fewer than a dozen foods have been scientifically proven to trigger acid reflux in all human bodies: mint oil, chocolate, deep-fried foods, alcohol, and coffee are on that list. Other triggers will be specific personally to you. That's why keeping a list of trigger foods is so important: it varies from person to person. Some digestive health experts do not believe that spicy food triggers acid reflux. Rather, they

believe spicy foods can intensify a person's symptoms if consumed during an acid attack. You be the judge. If you find that spicy triggers heartburn, put it on your list and stop eating it for a while, as you certainly won't be able to heal with prolonged exposure to foods that make you flux.

5. **Eat smaller portions more often throughout the day.** For those who enjoy eating, the really good news is you get to do it more often on the Acid Reflux Diet. By eating less more often, you will keep the contents of your stomach at a manageable level for your digestive system to process. Avoid the feeling of "too full" and "stuffed" at all costs. Think about breaking the food you eat each day into five different meals, all smaller than you'd normally eat: breakfast, mid-morning snack, lunch, mid-afternoon snack, and dinner. Sit down with friends and family for their scheduled meals—staying connected to others is an important part of human health—and then have two small meals of your own at mid-morning and mid-afternoon.

Within days or weeks of eating to beat back acid reflux, your symptoms should diminish in intensity and frequency. As you continue to keep stomach acid from fluxing into your esophagus, the cell lining will begin to heal. Once sufficiently healed, speak with your doctor about managing this chronic disease in the future.

Strategies for Acute vs. Chronic Symptoms

Acute symptoms are severe and appear suddenly, like a heart attack. The first time you experience acid reflux, you may experience acute symptoms that seemingly appear out of nowhere. You must see a doctor, even if your symptoms abate as quickly as they appeared. This may be a knock at the door by serious, chronic illness, so don't ignore it. If you bombard an acute attack with over-the-counter antacids, symptoms will diminish, but with continued use of non-prescribed antacids, you flirt with serious, long-term consequences. Over-the-counter acid reflux drugs can destroy healthy bacteria in the gut and set you up for long-term, recurring symptoms and disease.

A chronic condition develops over time and will not usually improve on its own. For example, osteoporosis is a chronic disease that can trigger an acute condition such as a broken bone. Your intervention is critical. Like osteoporosis and asthma, GERD is a chronic condition, and symptoms must be managed to ensure the best quality of life possible. Management leads to healing and good health but requires a doctor you trust and can work with over time.

The Acid Reflux Diet is aimed at slaying the chronic condition: if the diet is followed correctly, the symptoms that drag you down daily will soon run for cover and go into hiding.

Is the Acid Reflux Diet Right for You?

Q. Do you have acid attacks in your food pipe twice a week or more?

A. If you experience heartburn often (twice or more times a week) a doctor will diagnose you as a GERD sufferer. You will need to take medication and make food adjustments that keep stomach acid at home in the stomach, where it belongs. Ask your doctor to make sure the liquid surging from your stomach isn't actually bile from the liver, which will require a different treatment for similar symptoms. If those two essential strategies fail, your doctor might recommend surgery. Regardless, you have a chronic disease that must be managed correctly if you are to enjoy life and eat pain-free.

Q. I had a terrible attack of heartburn two weeks ago, but it hasn't returned. Should I be concerned?

A. You should be aware, not concerned. Most people suffer occasional bouts of heartburn during stressful times or while eating a trigger food, especially if they ate quickly. These occasional fluxes of acid should be treated with over-the-counter antacids for short periods of time (a day or two.) Using non-prescription antacids can kill good bacteria in the stomach that aids digestion, thus creating even more damage to the system that processes your food. Antacids may also cloak the severity of your symptoms, creating a false sense of health that will explode into reflux again and again.

Q. I can't live without a hamburger and fries. How can I follow this plan?

A. Simply put, you may not be ready for this diet if your desire for a hamburger overrides your desire to not feel absolutely horrible. If you enjoy being doubled over with pain and the urge to vomit, the Acid Reflux Diet is not for you. A hamburger and French fries can wait until you are healed, and that means fixing the way you eat, day in and day out. Once healed, an occasional hamburger is perfectly fine.

Q. Everyone tells me that exercise helps GERD, but my stomach is bloated and uncomfortable. What should I do?

A. A GERD sufferer should avoid high-impact exercise such as running and jumping. You want the low-impact activity of a good thirty-minute walk. Build up to it. Movement is crucial, but do not go for high intensity when you have chronic GERD symptoms, as bouncing and high impact will trigger acid movement in the food tube.

Q. How you eat is just as important as what you eat. Is that true?

A. The answer is yes, up to a point. Gulping down food is a destructive behavior when it comes to digestive health. Bacteria and acid in your stomach need time to do their work. If you rush the system, your food will back up, and the stomach will grind out more and more acid to break it down, setting you up for another acid attack. Slow down.

Be aware of every bite you take, chewing slowly and completely before swallowing.

Taste your food. If you can't describe in detail what you just put in your mouth and swallowed, you probably ate it too fast for healthy digestion.

Q. No day is the same. How can this diet be integrated into a busy life?

A. With calm intention and awareness, that's how. This is a time in your life when you need to stick up for yourself and build in time to heal. If you travel, try packing non-trigger foods that you can snack on. The same rules apply: Chew your food completely before you swallow, leaving time between bites until you are satisfied but not "full"—there's a difference. Pay attention and learn where that line (between satisfied and full) lies for you.

Q. Living with a large family means eating for the greatest common good. How do you ensure you are eating anti–acid reflux foods if you don't do the cooking?

A. Modern families are often made up of several generations with a wide array of needs, and that includes addressing health problems. You will need to sit the cook down and ask for help in treating your chronic disease. Have your list of trigger foods ready to hand over as you explain your situation. A true cook will relish the challenge. If you are the cook, well, no problem. Each meal needs to include foods that will sustain you without triggering attacks. Which fat the cook chooses as a cooking medium is as important as the choice to not serve a fatty cut of meat. Salt and sugar content matter as well. If frozen pizza is a staple, fresh vegetables, grains, fruits, and lean meat need to balance out the meal. Processed foods—commercially prepared and for sale in a grocery store—are often filled with unhealthy chemicals, too much sodium, and bad fats. While change is never easy, an entire family eating the Acid Reflux Diet way will be a healthy family indeed.

Q. When following the Acid Reflux Diet, what happens if you eat trigger foods?

A. Heartburn, probably. Just remember, every time you expose your LES to acid, you will damage whatever healing has taken place. And every time you damage it, you will experience symptoms for a longer period of time. If you have just begun the diet and eat a trigger food, you prolong your symptoms. If you've been on the diet successfully for a week or two, you may damage all the good healing work you've already done.

Q. How long does it take to heal GERD?

A. Everyone is different—but those that stick with the Acid Reflux Diet and medications prescribed by a doctor will have the best chances of a faster recovery. For others, the process can take years. For still others, the disease will rage on unchecked, eventually damaging the heart, destroying the esophagus's ability to function, and/or provoking the mutation of esophageal cells into cancer.

Q. Will changes in diet make grocery shopping difficult?

A. Believe it or not, many a diet has failed because of grocery shopping. Why? Endless choices entice and tempt. Don't fall for it. Turn left when you walk in the door of the supermarket if that's where the produce section is located. Don't wander around.

You'll shop in the following departments while on the Acid Reflux Diet: produce, meats, fish, dried grains, and beans. Don't lovingly stand in the potato chip aisle and drool. Get in and get out with whole foods. The Acid Reflux Diet should make grocery shopping easier and quicker.

Q. Can I drink sodas and sparkling water on the Acid Reflux Diet?

A. In a word: No. Here's why: Carbonation—the little bubbles in sparkling water and soft drinks—increases stomach distention to twice its usual size. Literally, you stretch your stomach with carbonation, and it expands to hold almost a gallon. Yup, that big stomach is big because of the bubbles that make you gurgle and burp. It's also pressing on your food pipe in that distended state, triggering a big attack of the acid that ruins your health.

Carbonation and anti-anxiety medications such as Zoloft and Xanax are often taken at bedtime for sleep. This combination is particularly potent for setting you up for a nighttime attack, ruining your sleep and your health over time.

CHAPTER THREE

Eating Well with Acid Reflux

Let's roll up our sleeves and get into the kitchen. This chapter is all about food, glorious food, the kind that heals acid reflux. This chapter will also talk about the foods that may hurt you, giving you a jump on your list of trigger foods to avoid.

As discussed earlier, acid reflux and GERD are no fault of yours. Modern life's stress, medications, and highly acidic foods wear down the gastro-intestinal system and loosen the esophageal sphincter (LES). A loose LES will cause acid splashes to come from the stomach. Acidic foods will damage the esophagus going down and as acid splashing up.

Processed foods are extremely dangerous to the GERD patient. The FDA requires commercially prepared foods to have more acid since it preserves food and allows products to remain on the shelves longer. Consumers are less likely to suffer a food-borne illness, but the acid works over time, shifting the danger from infection to chronic GERD disease.

The pH number tells you the acidity—or basic (alkaline)—nature of a food. For instance, distilled water has a pH of 7. The pH of the human body is quite close to distilled water—7.25 to 7.35. Therefore, the closer a food's pH is to the magic 7, the better. If a food has a pH lower than 4, an active sufferer of GERD should not eat it.

In addition to its effectiveness with GERD, the Acid Reflux Diet has been linked to promoting bone health, while a highly acidic diet increases chances of diabetes and heart disease.

The pH of Common Foods

Recently, medical researchers have found success treating drug-resistant GERD with only the Acid Reflux Diet. They discovered that acidic foods going down the food pipe can also contribute to the acidity level in the esophagus, damaging cells and loosening the LES. Turns out that food really matters.

Below is a list of common foods and their pH levels. What you read may surprise you, especially keeping in mind that when you begin the Acid Reflux Diet you'll be searching for foods with a pH of no less than 5. Any smaller number on the pH scale is too acidic for the GERD patient's gastrointestinal tract and will cause damage.

pH numbers will vary slightly from list to list because of many variables. One type of apple will register a lower pH than another kind of apple. In addition, conditions in the region where a food is grown affects acid levels as well. Don't split hairs. If a pH number's lowest range is below 4, set it aside. For example, peaches register pH in a range from 3.4 to 4.1. Unless you test every peach, you cannot know which one is above 4, so put this fruit aside until after you have done more healing.

Food	pH Level	Food	pH Level
apples	3.1–4.0	melons	5.7–6.7
asparagus	6.0–6.7	milk	6.4–6.8
avocados	6.27–6.58	oatmeal	6.2–6.6
bananas	4.5–5.2	olives, black	6.0–7.0
beans	5.4–6.6	olives, green	3.6–4.6
blueberries	3.12–3.33	oranges	3.69–4.34
broccoli	6.3–6.52	peaches	3.3–4.05
carrots	5.9–6.4	pickles, sour	3.0–3.4
cheese	5.1–5.9	potatoes	5.4–5.9
cherries	3.8–4.54	salmon	5.36–6.5
cranberry juice	2.3–2.52	sardines	5.4–6.6
egg whites	7.96	shrimp	6.5–7.0
egg yolks	6.1	soft drinks	2.0–4.0
ketchup	3.9	tomatoes	4.3–4.9
lemons	2.0–2.6	vinegar	2.4–3.4
limes	2.0–2.8		

The United States Food and Drug Administration (FDA) has come under attack in recent years over their food pyramid, which many feel promotes food manufacturers over human health. Despite your feelings on that subject, however, the FDA does have a comprehensive list of the pH balance of foods. Bookmark it and consult it often when planning your meals. Keep in mind that any pH number below 4 is not for you.

www.fda.gov

All alcohol—wine, beer, and spirits—tends to hover around a pH of 4 or lower. (Beer is listed anywhere from 2.5 to over 4). The best policy is not to guess—just avoid drinking it at the beginning of your diet. Coffee has a pH of around 4, and Coca-Cola is a whopping 2 on the pH scale. You need to drink thirty-two glasses of alkaline water to counter the acid in one Coca-Cola. Drinking alcohol is not advised in the first weeks of the Acid Reflux Diet, but it can be consumed in moderation during the maintenance phase, provided a drink does not trigger an attack.

In addition to the dangers of alcohol, juices, and soft drinks, the pH level of commercially bottled water varies as well. This one-hundred-billion-dollar-a-year industry makes products of varying acidity levels, and most public water systems will have a pH of around 7.

Since one of your tasks is to drink a lot of water between meals (not at meals, when it bloats the stomach), the list below may help. Watch the pH levels of sports drinks and energy drinks as well. The acid level is high, and dentists report damage to teeth. The beverage industry often disputes these numbers, so don't be surprised if you find wildly divergent pH numbers on certain products.

Beverage	pH Level	Beverage	pH Level
Aquafina	5.5	Nestlé Pure Life	7.3
Arrowhead	6.8	Pellegrino	4.0
Crystal Geyser	6.9	Poland Spring	7.2
Dasani	5.6	Propel Zero	3.5
Evian	7.9	Red Bull	3.3
Fiji	7.3	SmartWater	4.0
Gatorade	3.39	tap water	7.0
Glaceau FruitWater	4.0	Volvic	7.5

What to Stock in Your Pantry

Now that you understand the mechanisms that trigger acid reflux and painful GERD symptoms, you can begin to remove the foods that harm your health. The first place to start is the pantry. Stock the right fats for cooking and to use as dressings. This is one of the most important actions you can take, for in this way you will retrain your taste buds to register the flavors of real foods, instead of the mild taste of deep-fried fat.

Keep high-fiber, low-acid foods that don't spoil on hand: dried beans, whole-wheat pastas, and brown rice. Use dried herbs for flavor. Put aside—for now—salt and sugar. By examining and restocking the basics you use day in, day out, your health will change for the better. Once your health begins to change and you understand how good you can really feel, you'll grow stronger, faster, and more fit. Your life will be transformed by the change in your chemistry, physicality, and emotions.

As you begin the Acid Reflux Diet, go into "RR" mode: remove and replace in your pantry. Here's a list of what to take out and what to replace it with for maximum healing and health:

REMOVE

Bad fats: The first purge in your pantry should include all trans fats. Transfats were created in a laboratory by food scientists who added a hydrogen molecule to fat to keep it from spoiling on the shelves of markets. The result was so catastrophic for human health that the United States banned their use.

You'll find trans fats in commercially baked foods such as cookies, cakes, breads, crackers, margarine, bread crumbs, croutons, dressings, sauces, and pizza dough, as well as some fast foods and dairy products. Always check the label. If it says "partially hydrogenated," "shortening," or "margarine," don't use it. In fact, throw it out now.

Anything that contains more than 0.5 grams of trans fat per serving is dangerous to human health. Anything below that probably won't harm you.

REPLACE

Good fats: Run from that added molecule of hydrogen that turns fats into trans fats and instead use poly- and mono-saturated fats such as corn, olive, flaxseed, walnut, canola, peanut, and avocado oils when you cook and in dressings. PAM cooking spray has less than five calories and so little impact on the body that it's fine for you to use. It will help you cut down on calories as well.

Do not use saturated fats except for coconut oil. Coconut oil is a special type of saturated fat called medium chain triglyceride (MCT) that does not require acid bile to digest. In addition, coconut oil contains lauric acid, an antifungal, antibacterial, antiviral fatty acid found in mother's milk. You can buy both unrefined and refined coconut oil—but note that some coconut oil has partially hydrogenated fats, so be sure to read the label. Unrefined oil will be the mildest: heat exposure in refining makes the coconut flavor more pronounced, so if you do not want your food to taste of it, buy the unrefined variety.

REMOVE

Throw out all commercially processed foods: crackers and croutons, cookies and cakes, spaghetti sauces and dressings, and many boxed breakfast cereals. Start fresh—and by "fresh" that means whole foods—fruits, vegetables, lean meats, rice, beans, eggs, and fish. If you give your body a chance, in mere days it will no longer enjoy the chemicals you've been feeding it for years. Soon anything that isn't a whole food will taste false and unnatural.

Throw out soft drinks, sports drinks, and coffee, and hide the alcohol for at least two weeks. Drink tap water—in America, the pH is always around 7—in between meals if you can't find a low-acid bottled water. Put aside citrus juices and fruit juices such as cranberry. Your body is mostly water, and its pH is 7.35 to 7.45. Stay near to the 7-pH mark for hydration. This is important: you need clean water, close to your body's pH level, for optimal health.

For more information on how to eliminate caffeine in your diet, consult DrHyman.com, Internet home of pioneering physician Mark Hyman. He suggests eating a handful of seeds and nuts (almonds, pecans, walnuts, or pumpkin seeds) when craving caffeine—perhaps what you crave is really food. Drink one to three cups of green tea in the morning. Green tea's tiny amount of caffeine won't hurt you and just might ease the transition. Dr. Hyman also suggests supplements to assist your detox off caffeine, including taking a buffered 1000 mg of vitamin C at breakfast and dinner.

REPLACE

After you have thrown out the bad stuff, start stocking the good. Add packages of dried beans such as garbanzo, pinto, black, kidney, and soybeans, and grains such as quinoa, brown rice (pH of 6.2 to 6.7 instead of the slightly more acidic white), as well as the grains millet and kasha. Buy several types of nuts and seeds for snacking. Try almonds, walnuts, and pumpkin seeds. Do not stock your shelves with canned foods: pH levels are simply too varied and

Eating Well with Acid Reflux

often too high. For dried pastas, buy spinach and whole wheat, and serve with a white sauce. Red (or tomato-based) sauces are too acidic.

REMOVE

Remove condiments such as ketchup, vinegars, salt, sugar, mustard, pickles, citrus juices, sauces such as barbecue and salsa, green olives, and fermented and canned foods. All are too acidic for the Acid Reflux Diet, even in small amounts. Some condiments can be returned after the first two weeks of the diet, in healthy amounts, for occasional use.

REPLACE

For the Acid Reflux Diet, you will flavor your foods with fresh garlic, an alkaline food that also helps regulate the body's pH, lowers blood pressure, and battles heart disease. Flavored, healthy oils are used to drizzle on foods and add healthy fat, moisture, and taste. Dried herbs and spices will also enhance the flavor of fresh food in your new way of eating, at least for the first two weeks. Throw out old herbs and spices that have been sitting in your pantry, because these will have lost their taste. Use powdered and ground spices from the last six months and whole dried herbs from the past one to three years—anything older (or anything you don't remember when you bought) you should replace with new, fresher, more intense-tasting herbs and spices. You'll find yourself always more interested and satisfied by foods with different textures and flavor.

Cooking Methods and Equipment

The Acid Reflux Diet needs no special equipment or cooking gadgets: a functioning kitchen with clean water, heat, and an array of pots and pans will do fine. In fact, there is only one item to get out of the way.

Throw out the deep fryer, or put it in the garage. You will use the good fats to bake and sauté. Boiled, broiled, and simmered foods are great too. Invest in a simple steaming basket for vegetables and a wok to stir-fry foods in a small amount of peanut oil: it's easier than a frying pan to stir your ingredients.

If you are serving meals on large plates, try serving on smaller salad or dessert plates to control portion size. Remember, you are not going to stuff yourself at a single sitting. Your food intake is more frequent with smaller amounts of food passing through the esophagus into the stomach, where it digests rather than puts pressure on the food pipe, forcing up acid.

The Acid Reflux Diet requires that you hit the "pause" button when you eat, matching the speed of your intake more closely to the time it takes food to digest. So, after you finish preparation in the pantry, make sure to stop and enjoy your meal in the most peaceful, attractive spot you can find; only then will you learn to associate food with health, healing, and pleasure.

Tips on Dining Out

Dining out on the Acid Reflux Diet simply requires a little common sense. Don't go to a pizza joint if all they serve is pizza; you don't want the tomato-based sauce churning up acid. Don't think you can snack your way through the Fried Foods Festival with impunity—odds are, you'll pay.

Use your newfound knowledge of acid reflux when you eat out. Look at the menu. See all your trigger foods in bold print? This might not be the restaurant for you.

Patronize restaurants with larger, more diverse menus, and chances are you will find the right foods to eat. Avoid fast food—you'll probably eat it just as fast as they prepared it. The right restaurant will assist you in your efforts by accommodating your dietary needs and providing a good environment in which to consume your meals. If a restaurant tries to rush you out, that's as unhealthy for you as the wrong menu.

Most restaurants are categorized by the cuisine they serve. Stay out of the Chinese lunch buffet. Don't order "The Widower" curry, a Bindi dish in Grantham, England. The curry has twenty Naga Infinity chilis, creating six million Scoville units of heat. The dish is so hot that chefs wear goggles and a face mask to prepare it. In general, American, Italian, and Mediterranean foods are good cuisines for a night out. Also try restaurants that specialize in fish (not fried).

Portion sizes are also an issue. Some restaurants serve meals on platters you usually reserve for Thanksgiving Day. Don't eat this way—it's simply too much food. Make a deal with yourself that you will eat a quarter or half of the food on your plate and take the rest home. You can eat more in a couple of hours:

Eating time + food choices = a healthier digestive tract

Remember the formula above and you'll be on your way.

Ten Tips for Relieving Acid-Reflux Symptoms through Your Diet

1. **Don't Eat Foods on Your Trigger List.** The central purpose of the Acid Reflux Diet is to remove the foods that trigger acid rising in the food pipe. Use the FDA's online food acidity and alkalinity list. Pick foods with a pH of 5 or higher at the beginning, and you'll drop to eating 4's occasionally in your new lifestyle. Carry your list of trigger foods with you, and learn to note foods that irritate your system.

2. **Clean out your pantry and kitchen.** If you clean your pantry and refrigerator of trigger foods, as we described earlier, when you get a craving or need food quickly you won't reach for foods and ingredients that make you sick.

3. **Eat smaller meals more often.** For some people, this step is difficult. If you are consistently pressed for time and eating on the run, you must change. Slow down. Sit down. Don't eat your food in cars or at your keyboard. Stand up, go to a table, and eat. Enjoy what you put in your mouth and chew it slowly. Your physical and emotional state is important as well. Try—at all costs—to remove yourself from action so that you are calm as you eat.

   On the Acid Reflux Diet you'll have breakfast, a mid-morning snack, lunch, late-afternoon snack, and dinner. That's five small meals a day. If you need to tell family and colleagues that you are on a special dietary program, do it. If someone doesn't respect your desire to heal, well, that's their problem.

   In part, your five meals a day are designed to disrupt the routine of three large, regular meals. Disruption leads to awareness, and awareness to change.

4. **Do not lie down or sleep for two hours after eating.** When you flop on the couch after a big meal, you literally stop gravity from keeping your food where it belongs: the stomach. Sit upright. Don't take a nap or go to sleep for two hours after a meal. Don't eat in bed or while lying on the furniture. You'll find your sleep will improve as well.

5. **Self-test your reactions to foods.** Your condition will grow much worse if you do not attend to it. Buy pH strips and test your body's acidity and/or alkalinity. Test frequently: pH strips are available in many stores and cost between ten and fifteen dollars. Keep notes about

your pH level in relation to what you have eaten that day. Soon, you will become an expert on your own body chemistry and its reactions to certain foods. Note the pH of what has disturbed your system by consulting your favorite acidity/alkaline food chart. In short, pay attention to you.

6. **Food changes everything.** The effect of food on the human body is well documented. Today scientists have confirmed that when you change your diet you can alter your DNA into a healthier state. By eating the foods that are right for you, you change the life of the cells in your body. Their walls grow stronger and they improve their ability to cleanse themselves of toxins. Cells live longer if you treat them right. While moderating the level of acidity in your stomach, you'll notice a more stable emotional state as well. When you cut out additional sugars, your memory improves, and you won't experience as many mood swings or a physical "crash" after eating. Remove salt and you'll find that blood pressure lowers and bloating eases. All have an effect on how you feel emotionally as well as physiologically.

7. **Drink water—lots of it—with a pH of 7 or above.** You'll want to drink between a half gallon and a gallon and a half per day, depending on your level of activity and need. A gallon is the best amount to drink a day, if possible. Do not drink it with meals or you'll cause food in the stomach to expand. Instead, have a small glass of water with foods and then drink water in between.

   Just think of your gastrointestinal tract as a water park with a child who is stuck on the slide. A strong surge of water will discharge him into the pool, just as a surge of water helps discharge food into—and out of—the stomach.

   America's tap water is your best bet, as it usually hovers around 7 on the pH chart. If you have a favorite bottled water, look up its pH level. Do not drink carbonated water or soft drinks of any kind.

8. **Increase saliva production to help break down foods in the mouth.** If you rush eating your food, your mouth won't have time to help break it down properly. You also cannot process foods as well if you suffer from dry mouth (the medical term is "xerostomia"), which you may have developed from taking either over-the-counter or prescribed medications. To remedy this problem, chew gum about an hour before meals, avoiding mint (a trigger food) and focusing on soothing cinnamon and fruit flavors. You'll have lots of saliva when you sit down to eat.

9. **Lean on the good fats.** When you change the way you cook, you change the amount of fats you ingest. Substitute animal fats with olive, corn, or canola oils. Don't deep-fry foods: sauté in a tiny bit of clean oil or butter. Drizzle a little extra-virgin olive oil on foods as a dressing. Eschew margarine and all partially hydrogenated fats. Read labels, ask questions, get facts—your health depends on it.

10. **Drink raw aloe vera juice and slippery elm and chamomile teas.** Raw aloe vera juice is in many food and cosmetic products. Buy it and start slowly, because aloe relieves constipation, and you don't want to throw yourself immediately into diarrhea. At the same time, many GERD sufferers have constipation to start. Aloe vera levels the playing field so that you are eliminating waste at a speed that will aid digestion, not block it.

    Begin by drinking 1 ounce a day. Increase it to 2 ounces for a few days and then 3 ounces, provided you do not experience loose bowels. Build up to ½ cup several times a day. Aloe reduces acid levels in the stomach and heals skin cells burned by that acid. Either drink one to three times a day or twenty minutes before eating every meal.

    Slippery elm and chamomile teas soothe the mucus membranes of the gastrointestinal tract and might lessen your symptoms. Drink three to five cups a day, before meals, if possible. Tea will also keep the mouth busy when you might be pining for food. These teas will help you feel and digest better as well as you feel full. That full feeling will translate into weight loss, and any weight loss will help ease your reflux symptoms.

CHAPTER FOUR

Phase I: 14-Day Meal Plan

Now that you've absorbed all this information about your acid reflux, it's time to put it to work. Below you'll find a fourteen-day eating plan—Phase I of the diet—that will take you through the first two weeks of healing. During this period, you do not want to eat foods with a pH below 5. Afterward, you can graduate to Phase II—eating foods with a pH of 4 and above.

It's simple. In the first two weeks remove foods that may trigger an acid attack. Your pH level needs to be stabilized to the 7.35 to 7.45 region—the pH of human blood; anything above means your body is too alkaline and anything below is too acidic. Once you achieve a stable pH number within that narrow range, you can slowly add a greater variety of foods. Halting the flow of acid will heal the LES, and you should soon be able to return to beloved foods in moderation.

Remember: Some of the foods may upset your body chemistry despite registering a pH number in the correct range. You won't know until you follow the diet, make notes about your trigger foods, and remove anything that creates acid flux from your daily regime. After all, the driver of your health is you—you cannot expect a drug to do it all. A change in lifestyle is essential.

Eat your meals slowly, chewing your food carefully. Don't flop on the couch; stay upright and let gravity help you digest your food. Be aware and write down triggers.

Break apart your three main meals into five smaller ones, giving your stomach less food to process more completely. Move. Don't go to bed until two hours after eating, whenever possible.

If stress is part of your GERD equation, try meditation, guided imagery, hot baths, deep breathing, and exercise. Slow down. Be aware of your environment when you have an acid attack. What's going on? Who is around you? What medications are you taking and when? What are the most obvious things you can change to make your situation less stressful and more healing? All of these factors contribute to GERD, and you are the only one who can truly change the future of your health.

Most of the recipes that follow can be eaten in Phase I, and certainly in Phase II for the remainder of your life. Remember: Do not drink large quantities of fluids with your meals, as liquids cause the contents of the stomach to bloat. Instead drink plenty of water when you are not eating: your body needs it to function properly. In the morning, slowly wean yourself off coffee by decreasing the amount you drink and replacing it with green tea or decaffeinated black teas, which both contain small amounts of caffeine.

DAY 1 *Breakfast*: 1 cup Oatmeal with Nuts and Banana (47), ½ cup low-fat milk
Mid-morning snack: Savory Spinach Smoothie (45)
Lunch: No-Mayonnaise Tuna Salad (78); 1 whole-wheat pita, toasted and split in half, then in half again
Afternoon snack: ½ cup plain nonfat Greek yogurt mixed with 1 tablespoon honey, and a handful of raw almonds, sunflower seeds, or walnuts
Dinner: Pasta with Oil, Garlic, and Herbs (123), small side salad dressed with oil and a splash of fresh lemon, Mixed Summer Melons with Honey Cream (133)

DAY 2 *Breakfast*: Scrambled Eggs (50), 2 slices whole-wheat toast, buttered
Mid-morning snack: Spiced Nuts (61)
Lunch: Pumpkin (74) or Carrot Ginger Soup (73), Savory Bagel Chips (65)
Afternoon snack: carrot sticks, broccoli florets, cauliflower florets, Green Goddess Dressing (98)
Dinner: Perfect Fish (115), rice, Spinach Salad with Creamy Dressing (79), Avocado Pie (135)

DAY 3 *Breakfast*: Basic Granola (46); ½ cup low-fat milk
Mid-morning snack: Basic Non-Acidic Black-Bean Hummus (62), whole-wheat pita wedges
Lunch: Pear and Almond Sandwich (69), Honeydew Summer Soup (77)
Afternoon snack: banana with almond butter

Dinner: Individual Scotch Meat Loaves (121); Perfect Mashed Potatoes (104); baby spinach, boiled and drained with 1 tablespoon unsalted butter; Tropical Fruit Parfait (137)

DAY 4   *Breakfast*: 1 or 2 hard-boiled eggs, whole-wheat toast with unsalted butter, ½ cup plain low-fat Greek yogurt with almonds and 2 tablespoons honey
Mid-morning snack: baby carrots, broccoli, or cauliflower florets dipped in Creamy Dressing (79)
Lunch: sandwich: sliced cheese(s), alfalfa sprouts, and Creamy Dressing (79) on whole-wheat bread
Afternoon snack: soybeans, Crispy Chickpeas (100), or nuts
Dinner: Shrimp and Corn (119) on a bed of shredded lettuce; corn or rye bread with unsalted butter; Sweet Potato Wedges (63); Fluffy, Lemony Sweet Cheese Pudding (139)

DAY 5   *Breakfast*: ⅔ cup Basic Granola (46), ½ cup low-fat milk, 1 tablespoon honey
Mid-morning snack: No-Cook Banana Bites (68) or a banana and nuts
Lunch: large salad of butter, romaine, red leaf, or curly green lettuce; hearts of palm sliced into thin rounds; walnut pieces; and grated cheese with Creamy Dressing (79)
Afternoon snack: ½ whole-wheat or cinnamon bagel with unsalted butter, 1 tablespoon honey, or 2 tablespoons almond butter
Dinner: Turkey Burgers (84), Potato Salad (83), small salad of spinach or lettuce, Snickerdoodles (142)

DAY 6   *Breakfast*: Morning Sandwich (52)
Mid-morning snack: Banana Oat Smoothie (43), Stove Top Spicy Honeyed Almonds (67) or sunflower or pumpkin seeds with a pinch of salt
Lunch: any cream-based broccoli, potato, asparagus, or watercress soup; whole-wheat bread or pita, toasted
Afternoon snack: whole-wheat bagel, split and toasted; plain nonfat Greek yogurt; slices of cucumber; pinch of salt
Dinner: Fontina and Sage Grilled Cheese (90) sandwiches, Boiled Shrimp and Fresh Vegetable Platter with Green Goddess Dressing (98), Marshmallow Graham-Cracker Sandwiches (134)

DAY 7   *Breakfast*: Almond Butter and Banana French Toast (57); heavy cream whipped into stiff peaks, mixed with 1 teaspoon white sugar or 1 tablespoon honey
Mid-morning snack: Spiced Nuts (61), mixed nuts, or sunflower seeds
Lunch: Broccoli and Cheddar Cheese Soup (75) or another cream-based soup, small side salad
Afternoon snack: Layered Bean Dip (97) or low-sodium refried beans with extra-virgin olive oil and shredded cheese; toasted whole-wheat pita bread, cut into wedges
Dinner: Roasted Vegetables with Gruyère Cheese (111), brown rice, Vanilla Pudding (141)

DAY 8   *Breakfast*: Tropical Oatmeal (48) or any long-cooking oatmeal of your choice, ½ cup low-fat milk
Mid-morning snack: whole-wheat English muffins, toasted, with 2 tablespoons almond butter
Lunch: Lobster Roll (85); fresh vegetables on whole-wheat bread with fresh mozzarella, or any grilled fish or vegetable sandwich
Afternoon snack: banana, mixed nuts, or hummus and vegetables
Dinner: Roasted Vegetable "Pizzas"(114); avocado slices dipped in fresh lemon juice; 2 scoops low-fat vanilla frozen yogurt, sprinkled with chopped walnuts or pecans

DAY 9   *Breakfast*: any egg dish (not tomato-based), whole-wheat toast
Mid-morning snack: any smoothie in this book or any smoothie made with banana, mango, papaya, and/or coconut (no berry smoothies)
Lunch: any sandwich made of cheese and vegetables on whole-wheat or rye bread
Afternoon snack: carrots, broccoli, or cauliflower florets with Green Goddess Dressing (98)
Dinner: Roasted Fish on a Bed of Vegetables (117); pasta tossed in extra-virgin olive oil and 1 tablespoon grated Parmesan cheese; Fresh Figs, Almonds, and Manchego Cheese (140)

DAY 10   *Breakfast*: long-cooking oatmeal and ½ cup low-fat milk or any egg dish (without tomatoes)
Mid-morning snack: Sweet Bagel Chips (66), ½ cup low-fat vanilla Greek yogurt mixed with 1 tablespoon honey

Lunch: any sandwich recipe; Crispy Chickpeas (100), kale chips, or side salad

Afternoon snack: any smoothie, preferably with bananas, oatmeal, papaya, or mango (no berries)

Dinner: Stuffed Flounder (126) or simple grilled fish, brown rice, side salad, Vanilla Pudding (141) or ½ cup low-fat vanilla Greek yogurt mixed with 1 tablespoon honey and ¼ teaspoon cinnamon

DAY 11 *Breakfast*: any egg dish (without tomatoes) or granola with ½ cup low-fat cow, soy, or almond milk

Mid-morning snack: any toasted whole-wheat or rye bread with a melted slice of fontina, Gruyère, or Swiss cheese

Lunch: large main-dish salad of romaine, green-leaf, or butter lettuce with cooked eggs; sunflower seeds; sliced hearts of palm; shredded cheese; walnuts, pecans, or slivered almonds; shredded zucchini or carrot; and shredded cabbage, with Creamy Dressing (79) or Green Goddess Dressing (98)

Afternoon snack: banana with 1 tablespoon almond butter or ½ cup low-fat vanilla Greek yogurt mixed with granola or nuts

Dinner: Lentils and Kale (125), crusty whole-wheat breads, rice or small pasta dish, such as penne or bow-ties

DAY 12 *Breakfast*: oatmeal or Cream of Wheat Porridge (49) or any egg dish (without tomatoes)

Mid-morning snack: nuts, yogurt, and honey; or whole-wheat bread with 1 tablespoon almond butter

Lunch: Avocado-Egg Salad in a Whole-Wheat Wrap (127), small salad

Afternoon snack: smoothie made of low-fat milk or plain Greek yogurt (no berries)

Dinner: any grilled fish, Roasted Brussels Sprouts with Butter and Cheese (106) or Glazed Carrots (102) with rice, side salad, 2 scoops low-fat vanilla yogurt topped with Spicy Honeyed Almonds (67)

DAY 13 *Breakfast*: Sweet-Potato Hash with Eggs (122) or Simple Egg Casserole (55)

Mid-morning snack: banana and ½ whole-wheat English muffin with unsalted butter and nuts, or low-fat vanilla Greek yogurt stirred with honey and nuts

Lunch: any soup recipe in the book (or other cream-based soup of asparagus, broccoli, mushrooms, clam chowder, or fish stew—hold the bacon) or any sandwich recipe in the book
Afternoon snack: carrot sticks, cauliflower, or broccoli florets with cream- or bean-based dipping sauce
Dinner: Black-Bean and Portobello Mushroom Quesadillas (128); Guacamole (70); baked tortilla chips; Snickerdoodles (142) with frozen low-fat banana or vanilla yogurt

DAY 14 *Breakfast*: Simple Poached Eggs (56), whole-wheat toast, mixed cantaloupe and honeydew melon
Mid-morning snack: Cool Cucumber Soup (76)
Lunch: any sandwich recipe in the book
Afternoon snack: mixed nuts, Crispy Chickpeas (100), or lightly salted soybeans
Dinner: Roasted Vegetable Lasagna with Gruyère Cheese (113), side salad, Vanilla Pudding (141) with crumbled graham crackers sprinkled on top

PART TWO

Recipes for Phases I and II

Breakfast

CHAPTER FIVE

Breakfast

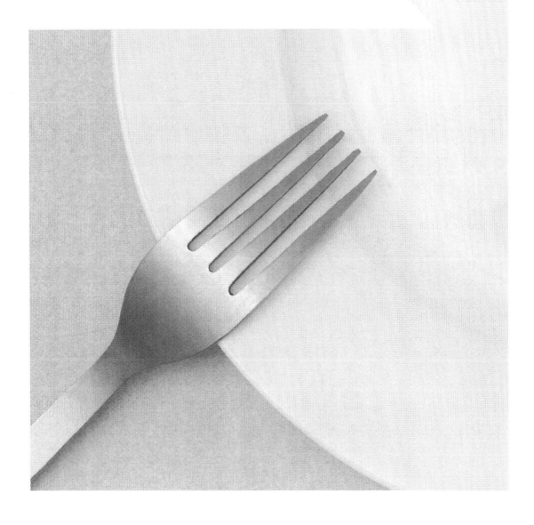

Banana Oat Smoothie

Sipping your breakfast—not gulping—is a great way to get your system going in the morning without having to cook. All the smoothies in this book have a perfect pH for your first two weeks of the Acid Reflux Diet. Always use plain low-fat yogurt, as sugar raises the acidity for a pH that is below 5. Cold ingredients make for better smoothies, so refrigerate or freeze bananas.

½ cup plain low-fat yogurt
¼ cup old-fashioned oats
½ cup low-fat milk
1 banana, frozen and broken into chunks
1 teaspoon honey
2 or 3 ice cubes

Put all ingredients into a blender and pulse until combined. Serve immediately.

Almond and Honeydew Smoothie

SERVES 1

2 cups chopped honeydew melon
1 cup almond milk
3 ice cubes
1 tablespoon honey

Put all ingredients into a blender and pulse until combined. Serve immediately.

Savory Spinach Smoothie

SERVES 1

1 cup spinach leaves, washed and stemmed
1 cup almond milk
2 teaspoons honey
2 or 3 ice cubes

Put all ingredients into a blender and pulse until combined. Serve immediately.

Basic Granola

This is the easiest of granola recipes. A small amount of sugar and salt is necessary for flavor, but it isn't enough to change the pH. If you like, add in new ingredients and change the taste of your granola. Try coconut flakes, swapping out the chopped nuts and seeds, or add bits of fresh fruit such as banana into individual bowls. Keep granola in a covered glass jar in your pantry.

3 cups long-cooking oats (not instant)
3 tablespoons light-brown sugar
1 teaspoon cinnamon
½ teaspoon salt
½ cup chopped nuts or seeds such as walnuts, almonds, pecans, and shelled sunflower seeds
⅓ cup honey
⅓ cup vegetable oil
1 teaspoon vanilla extract

Preheat the oven to 300°F.

In a large bowl, thoroughly mix all the dry ingredients—oats, sugar, cinnamon, salt, and nuts or seeds.

In a small bowl, whisk together the honey, oil, and vanilla extract. Pour over the ingredients in the large bowl and mix thoroughly.

Spread the oat mixture on a baking sheet and bake for 15 minutes.

Using a spatula, turn the granola over so that it browns evenly on the other side. Return to the oven and bake for 15 minutes.

Remove and let cool for 15 to 20 minutes. Serve with skim, almond, or coconut milk.

Oatmeal with Nuts and Bananas

SERVES 1

Either quick-cooking or old-fashioned long-cooking oats can be used in this recipe.

Quick oatmeal is cut in a way that traditional oatmeal is not, so it processes through the body more rapidly, causing the blood sugar to rise more quickly than it does with larger oats. The American Dietetic Society suggests that 1½ cups of oats per day lowers bad cholesterol, but don't eat that in one sitting. If you plan on reheating oats throughout the day to achieve this goal, use the longer-cooking kind.

1 cup quick-cooking or old-fashioned oats*
1 banana
¼ cup walnut pieces
½ teaspoon cinnamon
¼ to ½ cup low-fat or 2 percent milk

Prepare the oats according to the instructions on the package.

While the oats cook, peel and cut the banana into small, bite-size pieces.

Once cooked, put ⅔ cup oatmeal into a serving bowl. Sprinkle banana, nuts, and cinnamon over the top, and pour the milk over all. Serve immediately.

*Old-fashioned (long-cooking) and steel-cut oats will reheat better than instant oats. If you'd like to eat oatmeal as a snack later in the day, reheat in the microwave or on the stove top, adding tablespoons of water to moisten, if needed.

Tropical Oatmeal with Papaya and Coconut Milk

SERVES 2 TO 4

Oatmeal becomes more interesting with every ingredient you add to it. Here, the pH-friendly papaya and healthy coconut milk produce a tropical flavor to start your day.

This is a rich dish—decide if you want to include the butter it calls for during preparation. You won't need a great deal to get your motor started.

1 cup oatmeal
1 tablespoon butter
½ cup diced papaya
¼ cup coconut milk

Prepare the oatmeal according to the package instructions.

Stir the butter into the oatmeal, and spoon into serving bowls. Add the papaya on top and pour coconut milk over all. Serve.

Cream of Wheat Porridge

Porridge is known as oatmeal in the United States and Canada, but the word "porridge" is simply more poetic. Right now, Cream of Wheat has the perfect pH for your needs.

2 cups water or skim milk
1 cinnamon stick
⅓ cup Cream of Wheat
1 teaspoon sugar
½ cup skim, almond, or plain soy milk

If using water, pour into a medium saucepan over high heat, add the cinnamon, and bring to a boil. If using milk, pour into a medium saucepan over medium-high heat, add the cinnamon, and bring to a simmer but do not boil.

Add the Cream of Wheat to the pan and whisk out any lumps. Cook for 2 to 3 minutes or until the porridge has thickened.

Spoon into a serving bowl, sprinkle sugar on top, and add the milk. Serve.

Breakfast

Scrambled Eggs

Eggs (pH is 6.5) are a fabulous source of protein for the GERD sufferer and are delicious any time of day. Easy and quick to prepare, scrambled eggs are even tastier with add-ons—fold a couple of tablespoons of grated cheese, chopped vegetables, or a fistful of fresh herbs into the scramble and you'll discover it has a completely new character. Eggs are less moist out of the frying pan and perfect for sandwiches; cooked in the top of a double boiler, scrambled eggs are moist, delicate, and perfect alone on a plate.

1 tablespoon butter or a coating of cooking spray such as PAM
4 eggs
3 tablespoons low-fat or 1 percent milk
Pinch of salt

In a small frying pan or the top of a double boiler over medium, heat butter or cooking spray.

Crack the eggs into a medium or large bowl, then add the milk and salt. Beat with a fork or whisk until completely blended.

Add to frying pan or double boiler. Stir frequently, freeing cooked egg from the side of the pan so that liquid egg can flow beneath and cook. If you prefer moist eggs, remove from the pan as soon as the eggs are firm but still shiny. If you prefer your eggs dry—especially if you're making a sandwich—cook until the eggs lose that shine. Stir in any add-ons right before serving.

pH-Approved Add-Ons

- 1 or 2 tablespoons of shredded cheese

- ¼ cup chopped broccoli florets, asparagus, bell pepper, cooked mushrooms, or zucchini

- 2 tablespoons chopped herbs such as parsley, dill, or basil

Breakfast Crostini

SERVES 4

Crostini is an Italian creation that means "little toast" and is usually served with drinks or as an appetizer. However, it's perfect for morning. Pieces of toasted peasant bread are slathered with a variety of ingredients that will soothe your acid stomach.

Here, small balls of mozzarella cheese (bocconcini) marinating in water are split apart to mingle with herbs and olive oil.

1 pint of bocconcini, balls split in half
3 tablespoons extra-virgin olive oil
3 tablespoons chopped herbs, such as parsley and basil
Pinch of salt
2 garlic cloves
8 slices thick-crusted peasant bread, sliced thin and toasted

In a bowl, mix the bocconcini, oil, herbs, and salt. Cover and refrigerate overnight.

In the morning, remove and bring to room temperature.

Peel and split in half each garlic clove, and rub the cut surface over each slice of bread.

Slather cheese onto the toasted bread and serve.

Morning Sandwich

SERVES 2

For this breakfast, scramble eggs with your favorite add-ons in a frying pan, and tuck the finished dish into a whole-wheat pita pocket. Carry it outside, have a seat, and enjoy the fresh air as you eat. Breathe deeply.

Scrambled Eggs (page 50)
Whole-wheat pita pocket, split in half

Prepare Scrambled Eggs.

Split a whole pita in half to create two pockets.

Divide the eggs in half and spoon into the pocket of pita. Serve immediately.

Prevent Acid Reflux

Morning Egg Salad

Since commercial mayonnaise has a pH lower than 5, use some oil to moisten and hold the eggs together, then mound them on toasted pieces of whole-wheat bread. It's a bit different than mayonnaise-based salads but gives the same creamy satisfaction. Add lettuce to get in some more greens.

6 hard-boiled eggs, peeled and quartered
2 tablespoons extra-virgin olive oil
2 tablespoons heavy cream
Pinch of salt
¼ cup fresh parsley, chopped
4 slices whole-wheat bread
2 leaves of lettuce

Use the back of a fork to mash the eggs to desired consistency.

In a small bowl, whisk together the oil and cream. Add the salt and parsley and combine thoroughly.

Toast the bread, put a lettuce leaf on each of two slices, and mound high with the egg mixture.

Cover with the other slices of bread and serve immediately.

Breakfast

Simple Frittata

A frittata is a type of Italian omelet. You cook the eggs in a frying pan on the stove and finish the dish under the broiler. This final moment in the oven crisps the top of the eggs.

1 or 2 tablespoons butter
8 eggs
¼ cup low-fat or 2 percent milk
Pinch of salt
¼ cup grated cheese, such as Swiss, Gruyère, or white cheddar
½ cup cooked ground turkey
¼ cup chopped parsley

Preheat the broiler.

In a medium frying pan, melt the butter over medium heat.

While the butter melts, crack the eggs into a large bowl, and add the milk and salt. Use a fork or whisk to beat until all ingredients are combined.

Pour into the frying pan and cook as you would to scramble eggs, stirring often to loosen the cooked egg and let liquid egg flow beneath.

When the eggs are still moist but almost firm, add the cheese, turkey, and parsley, and fold into the eggs.

Slide the pan beneath your broiler and broil for 3 to 5 minutes, or until the top of the eggs are golden brown. Cool for 10 minutes, cut into wedges, and serve.

Simple Egg Casserole

This dish is all about keeping your pH alkaline, with eggs, cheese, spinach, and a pinch of cinnamon to help with inflammation. Frozen spinach needs to be taken out of the freezer and thawed, but otherwise, this is a quick dish that's easy to prepare. Additional egg whites are added to lower acidity even more and pump up the protein.

1 tablespoon canola oil, plus more for pie plate
3 large portobello mushroom caps, thinly sliced
6 eggs
1 cup low-fat milk
Pinch of salt
½ teaspoon cinnamon
¾ cup grated Gruyère cheese
1 (9-ounce) box frozen spinach, chopped, thawed, and drained

Preheat the oven to 350°F.

In a small or medium frying pan, heat the oil over medium-high. Add the mushroom caps and sauté for 3 to 4 minutes or until soft.

Remove from heat.

Crack three eggs into a large mixing bowl. Separate three more eggs, adding the whites only to the bowl. (Reserve the yolks for another use.) Add the milk and mix with a whisk or fork until combined. Add the salt and cinnamon and mix again, then add the cheese. Squeeze out as much moisture as possible from the spinach and add it to the bowl.

Use a paper towel to spread a little more canola oil over the bottom of a 9-inch glass pie plate. This will keep the eggs from sticking. Add the egg mixture.

Bake for 30 minutes or until the eggs firm up to your liking. Remove, cool for 10 minutes, and serve.

Simple Poached Eggs

Don't worry, the vinegar (too acidic for the first two weeks of the diet) does not actually change the pH of this dish to make it acidic: it merely holds the egg whites together in the almost-boiling water.

1 to 2 teaspoons rice vinegar
4 eggs
4 slices whole-wheat bread, toasted
Tiny pinch of salt

In a large skillet, bring 2 to 3 inches of water to a boil. Add the rice vinegar and decrease the temperature to medium. As soon as the bubbles disappear—this is just under the boiling point—crack an egg into a small cup and slide it into the water, using a spoon to keep the whites together.

Cover and cook, just under boiling, for 4 minutes. Remove the egg with a slotted spoon and drain on a paper towel. Repeat with the remaining eggs. Put each drained egg atop a piece of whole-wheat toast, sprinkling the top of each egg with the tiniest pinch of salt. Serve immediately.

Almond-Butter and Banana French Toast

Almond butter is an alkaline food and a great go-to for a boost of protein. Classic French toast with syrup must wait for later—the pH of maple is simply too acidic.

2 eggs
Dash of vanilla extract
4 tablespoons creamy almond butter
4 slices whole-wheat bread
1 banana, thinly sliced
3 to 4 tablespoons butter

In a medium bowl, beat the eggs with the vanilla.

Spread a thin layer of almond butter on each of the bread slices. Lay banana slices on top of two bread slices and cover with the remaining two bread slices to make two sandwiches.

In a large frying pan, heat the butter. Dip each sandwich in the egg mixture and add to frying pan. Cook each sandwich on one side until brown and then flip, cooking the other side until the egg is firm and the outside is cooked through. Serve immediately.

Snacks

Snacks

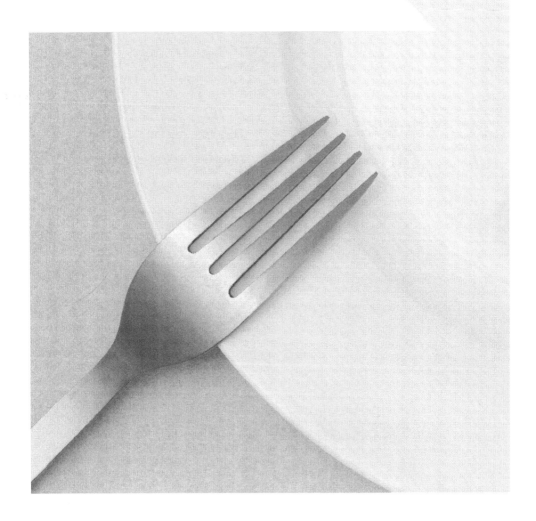

Spiced Nuts

Add healing spices to alkaline nuts for a perfect acid reflux–fighting snack.

3 cups mixed nuts, such as almonds, walnuts, pecans, and hazelnuts
3 tablespoons unsalted butter
½ teaspoon cumin
½ teaspoon ground cinnamon
3 tablespoons light-brown sugar
½ teaspoon salt

In a large, dry skillet over high heat, add the nuts and stir frequently, toasting lightly, for about 1 to 2 minutes.

Add the butter to the nuts and continue to mix until butter melts. Add the cumin, cinnamon, sugar, and salt, and continue to stir until nuts are coated. Remove from heat, spread across a sheet of aluminum foil, and let cool for 10 minutes. Serve.

Basic (Non-Acidic) Black-Bean Hummus

Cooked black beans are processed with oil and spices to make a bean paste that you can spread on whole-wheat pitas for a delicious, low-acid hummus. This mix will taste a bit different than store-bought hummus because we've taken out all the acid. A mere tablespoon of lemon juice will give you vitamin C without raising your acid levels, but this mix is not as salty as store-bought.

2 cups black beans, cooked
2 garlic cloves, chopped
2 tablespoons extra-virgin olive oil
1 tablespoon fresh lemon juice
½ teaspoon ground cumin
Pinch of salt
2 whole-wheat pitas, toasted and cut into wedges

Put all ingredients except pita into the bowl of a food processor and pulse until smooth. Remove and put into a serving bowl. Drizzle a little more olive oil on top, and serve immediately with toasted pita wedges.

Sweet Potato Wedges

SERVES 6

Sweet potatoes are healthy and pH friendly for the GERD patient; they don't spike your blood sugar as much as white potatoes do. Keep these around as a go-to slightly sweet, naturally satisfying food.

3 large sweet potatoes, peeled and cut into wedges
Cooking spray, such as PAM
1 teaspoon sugar
½ teaspoon salt

Preheat the oven to 500°F.

In a large bowl, spritz cooking spray over the top of sweet potatoes. Toss and spray again. Continue until all the potatoes are moist.

In a small bowl, mix together the sugar and salt and sprinkle over sweet potatoes. Toss to coat thoroughly.

Spread potatoes in a single layer on a baking sheet and bake for 10 minutes. Turn the potatoes, cook for 10 minutes more, and serve.

Snacks

No-Mayonnaise Deviled Eggs

Mayonnaise is acidic, so use plain low-fat Greek yogurt for this recipe instead. (As you progress in your healing, you'll be able to add the mayonnaise back in.) We suggest adding lemon peel to perk up the flavor, but if you are just beginning the diet, skip it and stick with the lemon juice. Note that these deviled eggs make a great portable snack; to take with you, simply put the egg halves back together and wrap in plastic or foil.

6 hard-boiled eggs, peeled and sliced in half
1 tablespoon finely chopped parsley
Zest of ¼ lemon
2 tablespoons plain low-fat Greek yogurt
1 teaspoon lemon juice

Using a fork, tease out the cooked yolk in each egg. Put egg yolks in a bowl, and place the twelve egg halves on a platter.

Add the parsley, lemon zest, yogurt, and lemon juice to the bowl, and use the back of a fork to mash all ingredients.

Using a spoon, gently pack each egg half with the yolk mixture. Arrange on a platter and serve immediately.

Savory Bagel Chips

SERVES 3 OR 4

Set out whole-wheat bagels overnight so that they turn stale, and slice them thin. Toast and cover with savory or sweet flavors, depending on your mood.

3 stale whole-wheat bagels, thinly sliced
2 or 3 tablespoons unsalted butter, melted
2 garlic cloves, minced

Toast the bagel slices until they are light brown.

In a small saucepan over low heat, melt the butter, add the garlic, and cook for 1 minute.

Remove from heat, and brush butter onto the bagel rounds. Serve immediately.

Sweet Bagel Chips

This is a sweet version of bagel chips with lots of cinnamon to soothe your stomach after the first two weeks of the Acid Reflux Diet. Remember to set the bagels out uncovered the night before so that they become stale.

3 stale cinnamon-raisin bagels, thinly sliced
2 to 3 tablespoons unsalted butter, melted
2 tablespoons sugar
½ teaspoon cinnamon

Toast the bagel slices until they are light brown.

In a small saucepan over low heat, melt the butter, add the sugar and cinnamon, and stir for 30 seconds to 1 minute. Remove from heat, and brush butter on the bagel rounds. Serve immediately.

Stove Top Spicy Honeyed Almonds

SERVES 3 OR 4

Smoky sweet, this will become a snack staple whenever you need to manage your GERD symptoms after the first two weeks of your diet. Omit the chili powder if you feel it's one of your triggers.

1½ cups raw, unblanched almonds
2 teaspoons sugar
2 to 3 tablespoons honey
½ teaspoon salt
¼ teaspoon ground cumin
½ teaspoon chipotle chili powder

In a large frying pan over medium-high heat, toast almonds, stirring frequently, for 5 to 6 minutes.

In a small ceramic or glass bowl, combine the sugar, honey, salt, cumin, and chili powder, and microwave on high for 30 seconds. Alternatively, empty the mixture into a small saucepan, and heat over medium-high for 2 to 3 minutes.

Add the warm honey mixture to the almonds in the frying pan. Cook for 2 minutes more, stirring constantly to coat.

Spread the almonds over a long sheet of wax paper, breaking apart any clumps. Let cool and dry, and serve.

No-Cook Banana Bites

So simple, you can do it with your eyes closed. Banana chunks are dipped in yogurt and rolled in nuts for a power snack that soothes the acid damage in your food tube.

1 cup low-fat vanilla yogurt
2 firm bananas, cut crosswise into ¾-inch slices
½ cup almonds, walnuts, or pecans, chopped

Spoon the yogurt into a small bowl. Spread the chopped nuts on a plate. Dip a banana slice into the yogurt, then roll in the nuts. Place on a plate or baking sheet covered with wax paper. Repeat until all bananas are dipped. Put in the freezer for at least 30 minutes. Serve.

Pear and Almond Sandwich

Get to know almond butter: it is alkaline whereas peanut butter is slightly acidic. Almond butter has 25 percent less saturated fat than peanut butter, 26 percent more vitamin E, 3 percent more iron, and 7 percent more calcium.

5 tablespoons almond butter
4 slices whole-wheat bread, toasted
2 pears, split, cored, and thinly sliced

Spread almond butter on each slice of bread; cut each slice in half.

Lay pear slices on top of the almond butter and serve.

Guacamole

Avocados register as a mid-6 on the pH scale and are a soothing food for the GERD sufferer. Red onions are much less acidic than white and can be eaten in the first two weeks of the diet, while the lime juice in this recipe is too scant to have much effect on the pH scale.

2 tablespoons chopped red onion
2 teaspoons fresh lime juice
⅛ teaspoon salt
1 garlic clove, finely minced
1 ripe avocado, peeled
2 tablespoons chopped cilantro leaves

Put all ingredients into a food processor, and pulse until guacamole is smooth with small chunks throughout. Serve with toasted whole-wheat pita wedges, carrot sticks, broccoli, bell pepper, or cauliflower.

Soups, Salads, and Sandwiches

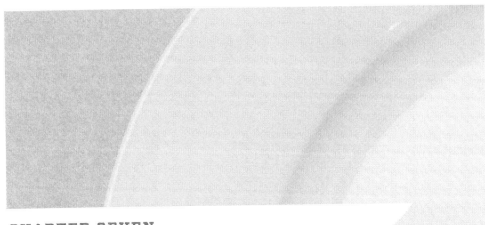

Soups, Salads, and Sandwiches

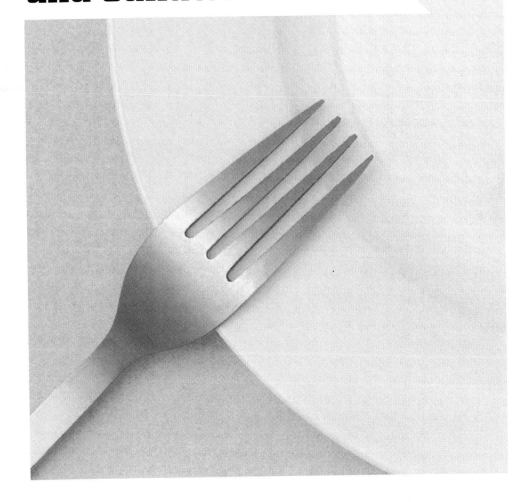

Carrot Ginger Soup

This soup is for the second phase of the Acid Reflux Diet, as the sour cream is slightly acidic. If this recipe appeals to you, try it. It may not trigger any adverse effects even in the first phase—it all depends on your individual chemistry. As always, don't continue eating it if you experience acid splash-back.

1 tablespoon unsalted butter
½ white onion, chopped
3 cups low-sodium, fat-free vegetable broth
1 pound baby carrots, peeled
1 tablespoon grated fresh ginger
3 tablespoons fat-free sour cream, for garnish
3 tablespoons chopped chives, for garnish
½ teaspoon salt

In a large saucepan or medium stockpot, melt the butter over medium heat. Add the onion and cook, stirring frequently, for 6 minutes or until soft and translucent.

Add broth, carrots, and ginger. Increase the heat to high and bring to a boil. Reduce the heat and simmer the soup for 30 minutes. Remove from heat and let cool slightly.

Using an immersion blender or a food processor, pulse the soup until smooth. Return to the stove over medium heat until the soup is warmed through. Ladle into bowls. Top with a tablespoon of sour cream, and sprinkle with chives as a garnish. Season with salt and serve.

Pumpkin Soup

Pumpkin, milk, and cinnamon are part of an acid-reflux soother of the highest order. This soup is low-fat and creamy as well.

¾ cup water
½ small onion, chopped
1 (15-ounce) can pumpkin purée
2 cups unsalted vegetable broth
½ teaspoon ground cinnamon
½ teaspoon nutmeg
1 cup fat-free milk

In a medium saucepan over high heat, bring ¼ cup of the water to a boil. Add the onion and boil until soft and tender, about 3 minutes. Keep the onion moist throughout, adding a tablespoon of water at a time if necessary.

Add the remaining ½ cup water, the pumpkin, broth, cinnamon, and nutmeg.

Bring to a boil, then reduce heat and simmer for 5 minutes. Add the milk and continue cooking until the soup is warmed through. Serve.

Prevent Acid Reflux

Broccoli and Cheddar Cheese Soup

Cheese and broccoli are perfect foods for the acid-reflux patient at any phase.

Cooking spray, such as PAM
3 tablespoons chopped onion
2 garlic cloves, minced
4 cups low-sodium chicken broth
3 cups broccoli florets
3 cups reduced-fat milk
⅓ cup flour
8 ounces grated mild white or yellow cheddar

Spritz the bottom of a large saucepan with cooking oil, and heat over medium-high.

Add the onions and garlic and sauté for 3 minutes.

Add the broth and broccoli, bring to a boil, and reduce the heat to a simmer. Cook for 10 minutes.

In a medium-sized bowl, combine the milk and flour, whisking until completely blended. Add to the saucepan and cook, stirring constantly, for 5 minutes or until thickened.

Add the cheese and stir until melted. Using an immersion blender or a food processor, pulse one-fourth of the soup only. Return to the pan, stir, and serve.

75

Soups, Salads, and Sandwiches

Cool Cucumber Soup

In Phase II of the Acid Reflux Diet, this cooling soup will be a go-to dish for summer—it also tastes great in fall and winter.

3 cups plain Greek yogurt
1½ cups low-fat, low-sodium vegetable broth
2 English cucumbers, peeled and diced
4 green onions, white and green parts thinly sliced
2 tablespoons chopped parsley leaves
2 tablespoons chopped dill
Juice of ½ lemon
Pinch of salt

In a large bowl, whisk the yogurt and broth until blended.

Using a food processor, purée 1 cucumber, 2 sliced green onions, parsley, and dill. Add to the yogurt-broth mixture and whisk until blended. Add the remaining cucumber and green onions, and whisk. Refrigerate for at least 1 hour, and serve, garnishing with lemon juice and seasoning with salt.

Honeydew Summer Soup

Perfect for Phase I or II of the Acid Reflux Diet, this cooling soup will soothe the food tube and is perfect for snacks. Notice how good it feels as it slides into your stomach. Try it with cantaloupe or other melons as well.

4 cups cubed honeydew melon
2 teaspoons lime juice
1 tablespoon honey
1 cup nonfat vanilla yogurt

Put all ingredients into the bowl of a food processor and pulse until smooth.

Refrigerate for at least an hour and serve with another spoonful of yogurt as a garnish.

No-Mayonnaise Tuna Salad

Since mayo is acidic, try this way of making tuna salad throughout the course of eating for acid reflux. Make sandwiches with whole-wheat breads and pitas and a leaf of lettuce for crunch.

1 (5-ounce) can tuna, preferably wild, packed in water or olive oil
1 celery stick, finely diced
¼ cup plain nonfat Greek yogurt

Drain the tuna and empty into a bowl. Add the celery and yogurt and mix thoroughly.

Add-ins:

Phase I:

- ¼ cup minced apple

- 1 tablespoon minced parsley

- ¼ cup walnuts, lightly toasted

Phase II:

- ¼ cup minced red onion

- 1 tablespoon chopped sour pickle

- 1 tablespoon chopped dill

Spinach Salad with Creamy Dressing

SERVES 4

Spinach is a mild food, ideal for acid-reflux sufferers, and packed full of nutrients. Served with a yogurt-based dressing, this salad is perfect for all your efforts to stop GERD.

For the salad
2 tablespoons chopped red onion
4 hard-boiled eggs, peeled and cut into quarters
1 (11-ounce) package spinach, picked over and stems removed

For the Creamy Dressing
1 (8-ounce) container plain low-fat yogurt
1 teaspoon fresh lemon juice
2 teaspoons prepared Dijon mustard
2 teaspoons chopped chives
2 teaspoons chopped parsley

To make the salad: In a large bowl, gently mix the onion and eggs into the spinach.

To make the dressing: In a small bowl, whisk the yogurt, lemon juice, mustard, and herbs until completely combined. Pour over salad as desired.

Old-Fashioned Steak-House Lettuce Wedge with Blue Cheese Dressing

SERVES 1

This is how America made salads in the 1960s—it's low-acid and old-school.

¼ head iceberg lettuce
1 red onion, thinly sliced and separated into rings
1 hard-boiled egg, chopped
¼ cup crumbled blue cheese
Creamy Dressing (page 79)

Put the lettuce wedge on a plate.

Lay the onion rings over the wedge, and sprinkle chopped egg over all.

Crumble the blue cheese into the Creamy Dressing. Drizzle on the wedge and serve.

Waldorf Salad, Hold the Mayo

SERVES 2

This has all the ingredients to promote health. When you replace acidic mayonnaise with yogurt, you can expect a fresher flavor than those old-style, mayonnaise-soaked Waldorf salads.

4 apples, peeled, cored, and chopped
2 stalks celery, thinly sliced
½ cup walnuts, chopped
½ cup plain nonfat Greek yogurt
1 teaspoon sugar
1 teaspoon lemon juice
Dash of salt

In a large bowl, combine the apples, celery, and walnuts.

In a smaller bowl, whisk together the yogurt, sugar, lemon juice, and salt. Pour over apple mixture, chill for at least 30 minutes, and serve.

Salad of Mixed Baby Greens with Alkaline Add-Ins

Prepackaged baby greens are the perfect base for a large or small salad for lunch or an afternoon snack.

For the salad
1 (5-ounce) package baby lettuces
¼ cup crumbled or shredded cheese of your choice
Handful of walnuts or pumpkin or sunflower seeds

Add-ins
¼ cup thinly sliced hearts of palm
¼ cup thinly sliced asparagus
¼ cup drained kidney, black, or lima beans
¼ cup chopped avocado
1 hard-boiled egg, peeled and coarsely chopped
Handful of cooked shrimp
¼ cup diced drained tofu
Handful black olives, sliced
¼ cup fresh corn kernels

For the dressing
2 to 3 tablespoons extra-virgin olive oil
1 teaspoon fresh lemon juice
Dash of salt
3 tablespoons chopped parsley, dill, or cilantro

To make the salad: Put the lettuce, cheese, and nuts or seeds into a large bowl. Mix in add-ins of your choice.

To make the dressing: In a small bowl, combine the oil, lemon juice, and salt, and whisk until completely blended. Add the herbs and stir. Drizzle over the lettuce and serve.

Potato Salad

Potatoes come in at close to 5 on the pH scale. Perfect for the second phase of the diet, this potato salad makes a fabulous lunch or afternoon snack.

For the salad
2 red potatoes, boiled, skinned, and cubed
1 stalk celery, thinly sliced
1 green onion, white and green parts sliced thin
2 tablespoons chopped red onion

For the dressing
¼ cup plain nonfat Greek yogurt
½ teaspoon lemon juice
½ teaspoon sugar
Pinch of salt
2 tablespoons chopped parsley

To make the salad: In a large bowl, gently mix together potatoes and remaining ingredients.

To make the dressing: In a small bowl, whisk together the yogurt and lemon juice. Add the sugar, salt, and parsley, and continue to whisk until completely combined.

To assemble the salad: Pour the dressing over the potatoes, mix carefully, and serve.

Turkey Burgers

Turkey surfs the pH line between alkaline and acidic. Buy the best ground turkey—white meat only—available, and the pH of this recipe will be high enough for the first phase of the Acid Reflux Diet.

½ pound ground white-meat turkey
1 egg, beaten
¼ teaspoon ground sage
1 to 2 tablespoons vegetable oil
2 whole-wheat English muffins
½ cup plain nonfat Greek yogurt
Juice of ½ lemon
4 romaine, butter, or iceberg lettuce leaves

In a medium bowl, thoroughly mix ground turkey with beaten egg and sage.

Heat the oil in a skillet over medium-high. Divide the turkey mixture in two, and form two patties. Add to skillet and cook through.

Toast the English muffins.

In a small bowl, whisk the yogurt and lemon juice until combined. Slather on each side of the toasted, split English muffins.

Put a leaf of lettuce on one side of each English muffin, then add a turkey patty, and follow with another lettuce leaf. Top with the other half of the muffin and serve.

Lobster Rolls

Lobsters remain a strong catch for fishermen, and almost every supermarket of any size in America will have them for sale in a tank. The supermarket personnel will usually cook lobsters for you, so the squeamish won't have to put them in a pot at home. This sandwich is fine for either phase of the diet.

2 large lobsters, cooked and meat removed from shell
½ stick unsalted butter, melted and slightly cooled
1 tablespoon mayonnaise
1 teaspoon fresh lemon juice
½ teaspoon salt
2 tablespoons chopped parsley
2 top-loading hot dog buns

In a large bowl, thoroughly combine lobster meat and butter.

Add the mayonnaise, lemon, salt, and parsley and mix again. Divide the lobster mixture between 2 top-loading hot dog buns and serve.

Soups, Salads, and Sandwiches

Avocado and Cheese on Nutty Whole Wheat

SERVES 2

Avocado is a rich treat that's perfect for the food pipes and stomachs of acid-reflux patients—it's creamy and full of great nutrients and good fats. If you need a healthy snack at any point in the diet, try slices of avocado dipped in lemon juice with a dash of salt.

4 slices Swiss cheese
4 slices nutty whole-wheat bread
¼ cup plain Greek yogurt
1 tablespoon mayonnaise
¼ teaspoon salt
1 ripe avocado, peeled, pitted, and thinly sliced
½ cup alfalfa or other sprouted seeds

Place a slice of cheese on each piece of bread.

In a small bowl, whisk together yogurt, mayonnaise, and salt. Slather this mixture on each slice of cheese on the bread.

Lay slices of avocado on top of the yogurt mix, and mound sprouts on top of the avocado. Top with the other slice of bread. Cut the sandwiches in half, and serve immediately.

Mozzarella and Basil Sandwich

This simple sandwich of cheese, oil, and herbs has sustained many, and the pH is especially low. If you are in Phase I, do not add the tomato—this sandwich is still delicious without it. (You can add a generous slice of tomato in Phase II.) Be sure to use a peasant bread with a nice, thick crust.

8 slices mozzarella cheese
4 slices white peasant bread, toasted light brown
¼ cup fresh basil leaves
2 tablespoons extra-virgin olive oil
Dash of salt
2 thick slices of tomato (Phase II only)

Lay two slices of mozzarella cheese on each piece of bread. Pile up basil leaves on the cheese and drizzle with oil. Salt lightly.

If you are in Phase II, add a tomato slice to one side of each sandwich.

Cover with two remaining slices of bread and serve.

Broccolini and Egg Sandwiches

SERVES 2

Broccolini is an interesting vegetable, and this is a splendid, low-acid sandwich. Branch out—try new vegetables. Battling acid is an excellent time to explore new foods that don't irritate.

3 tablespoons extra-virgin olive oil
2 to 3 bunches broccolini
2 garlic cloves, chopped
2 tablespoons unsalted butter
4 eggs
2 to 3 tablespoons low-fat milk
Dash of salt
2 slices provolone cheese
Half a baguette, split in half, each half split open

In a large skillet, heat olive oil on high until hot. Add the broccolini and garlic, and stir until soft, 4 to 5 minutes. Remove and set aside.

In a small skillet, melt the butter over medium heat. In a small bowl, beat the eggs with the milk and salt, and pour into the skillet.

Cook, stirring frequently, until the eggs are firm.

Add the broccolini mixture and cheese to the pan and stir. Mound half of the mixture in one split baguette and half in the other. Serve.

Gruyère Cheese, Apple, and Fig Sandwich

Gruyère is one of the great melting cheeses. Combine with two types of fruit and toast for an extraordinary Phase II sandwich. Look for figs in season: the pH makes the fruit great for snacking in either phase of the diet.

4 slices (½ cup shredded) Gruyère cheese
4 slices whole-wheat bread
1 firm, tart apple, cored and thinly sliced
4 figs, chopped or thinly sliced
2 to 3 tablespoons butter

Add cheese to the top of two bread slices, followed by apple slices and figs.

Close the sandwich with the remaining two bread slices.

In a frying pan over low heat, melt the butter. Carefully place one sandwich in the butter and cook for 2 to 3 minutes. Turn over and cook for 2 to 3 minutes more until the cheese is melted and the fruit is warm. Repeat with the second sandwich, adding more butter if needed. Serve immediately.

Fontina and Sage Grilled Cheese

SERVES 2

A great melting cheese, fontina mingles here with fried sage, making for a flavorful grilled sandwich with a more sophisticated taste than the average grilled cheese.

4 slices fontina cheese
4 slices whole-wheat bread
2 to 3 tablespoons butter
8 fresh sage leaves

Lay the slices of fontina on two slices of bread.

In a large skillet, melt half of the butter. Add the sage leaves and fry for several minutes.

Remove and divide among the bread slices.

Top with the remaining two slices of bread.

In the same skillet, melt the remaining butter over low heat. Place the sandwich in the butter and cook for 1 to 2 minutes on one side, pressing the sandwich together with the back of a spatula. Turn over and cook for another 2 to 3 minutes. Serve immediately.

Mushroom and Manchego Cheese Sandwich

Vegetables and cheese make for a great sandwich. Mushrooms are low in pH, so if you prefer, substitute them with the same amount of coarsely chopped zucchini.

3 tablespoons unsalted butter
½ cup white button mushrooms, sliced
½ cup cremini mushrooms, sliced
½ cup oyster mushrooms, sliced
Pinch of salt
Pinch of sugar
4 slices whole-wheat bread
½ cup shredded Manchego cheese

In a large frying pan over medium heat, melt half of the butter.

Add the mushrooms, salt, and sugar to the pan. Stir and cook for 8 to 10 minutes or until the mushrooms are soft and have released their moisture. Remove from heat.

Pile mushrooms on two slices of bread. Top with Manchego cheese and cover with the remaining slices of bread.

Add the remaining butter to the pan, and melt over medium-high heat. Place the two sandwiches in the pan and cook, pressing each sandwich together with the back of a spatula, for about 2 minutes. Flip the sandwiches, cook for another 2 minutes, and serve.

91

Soups, Salads, and Sandwiches

Fresh Veggie Bagels

Fresh vegetables work for both phases of the diet, but tomato (a fruit) can only be eaten—in moderation—in Phase II. Add the tomato if you have reached the third week of your new eating plan.

2 whole-wheat bagels, sliced in half
1 tablespoon yellow mustard
2 romaine lettuce leaves
½ cucumber, thinly sliced
1 red bell pepper, cut into 1-inch strips
2 thick slices tomato (Phase II only)
½ cup sprouts

Toast the bagels.

Slather mustard on each bagel slice, top with lettuce, cucumber, pepper, tomato (Phase II), and sprouts. Top with remaining bagel slices and serve.

Chickpeas in Whole-Wheat Pitas

SERVES 2 TO 4

In some parts of the world, chickpeas provide a great deal of nutrition and fiber to local diets. Here, we process with cucumbers and herbs for a delicious chickpea purée on whole-wheat pitas. If you use canned chickpeas, be sure to rinse several times in water to remove all the salty moisture.

2 garlic cloves, minced
5 tablespoons plain, nonfat Greek yogurt
1 tablespoon reduced-fat mayonnaise
1 tablespoon lemon juice
2 cups cooked chickpeas (garbanzo beans)
1 tablespoon chopped dill
1 large carrot, peeled and shredded
4 whole-wheat pitas
4 romaine or curly green leaf lettuce leaves

In a bowl, thoroughly mix the garlic and 4 tablespoons of the yogurt.

Put the yogurt mixture, mayonnaise, lemon juice, and chickpeas into the bowl of a food processor and pulse until smooth.

Remove to a medium bowl. Add the dill and stir.

In a small bowl, mix the carrots with the remaining 1 tablespoon of yogurt.

Split the pitas and stuff a lettuce leaf inside each. Divide the chickpea mixture between the pitas, then add the carrot and yogurt mixture. Serve.

CHAPTER EIGHT

Appetizers and Side Dishes

Layered Bean Dip

Boiled Shrimp and Fresh Vegetable Platter with Green Goddess Dressing

Potato and Cheese Phyllo Squares

Crispy Chickpeas

Almost Tzatziki

Glazed Carrots

Broccoli and Cheese

Perfect Mashed Potatoes

Delicious Cabbage

Roasted Brussels Sprouts with Butter and Cheese

Creamed Corn

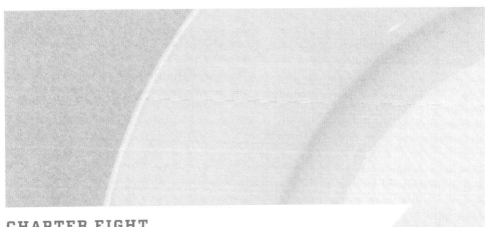

Appetizers and Side Dishes

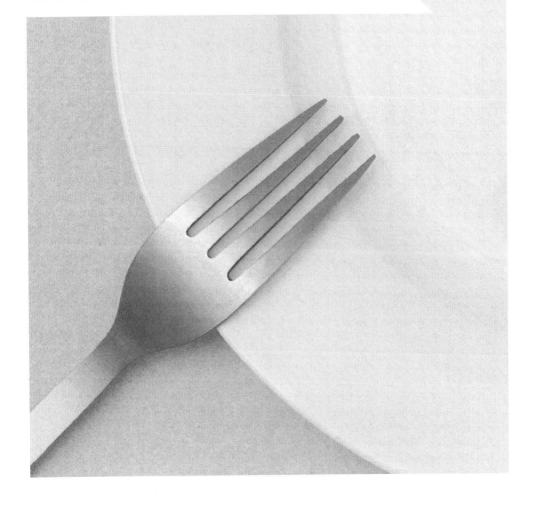

Layered Bean Dip

A take on the popular American dip, this takes out the extremely acidic ingredients without compromising the experience. Serve with baked tortilla chips or whole-wheat toasted pita slices. Omit the tomato if you are in Phase I.

2 cups homemade (one 15-ounce can) refried beans
1 tablespoon extra-virgin olive oil
½ teaspoon chipotle or plain chili powder
¼ teaspoon ground cumin
1 avocado, peeled, pitted, and chopped
1 tomato, cut in half, pulp and seeds squeezed out,
    chopped (Phase II)
2 teaspoons lime juice
Dash of salt
⅓ cup plain Greek yogurt
⅓ cup black olives, pitted and sliced
¼ cup chopped cilantro leaves

In a small saucepan over medium-high heat, warm the refried beans, stirring in the olive oil, chili powder, and cumin.

As soon as the beans are warmed through, spread them on the bottom of a medium-sized glass serving bowl.

Spread the avocado chunks over the beans and spread the tomato (if using) over the avocado.

In a small bowl, whisk the lime juice and salt into the yogurt and spread over the tomato (if using) or the avocado (if in Phase I).

Sprinkle the olives on top, followed by the chopped cilantro. Serve with baked tortilla chips or whole-wheat pita.

Boiled Shrimp and Fresh Vegetable Platter with Green Goddess Dressing

For the dressing

1 cup plain low-fat Greek yogurt

½ cup finely packed parsley leaves

1 green onion, white and green parts thinly sliced

2 tablespoons chopped dill

1 tablespoon chopped tarragon

2 teaspoons lemon juice

2 garlic cloves

½ teaspoon salt

1 pound freshly boiled shrimp, shells on

1 cup baby carrots, peeled

1 cup bite-size broccoli florets

1 cup bite-size cauliflower pieces

To make the dressing: Put all ingredients into the bowl of a food processor and pulse until creamy and flecked with bits of green. Pour into small serving bowl and refrigerate for at least 30 minutes.

Place the dressing in the center of a large platter, and pile shrimp and vegetables around it. Serve.

Prevent Acid Reflux

Potato and Cheese Phyllo Squares

This Greek dish is a simple appetizer made with frozen phyllo from the grocery store.

Melted Gruyère cheese on a potato provides heavenly satisfaction for the acid-reflux patient in either Phase I or II.

8 fingerling or Dutch potatoes
1 sheet frozen phyllo dough, thawed
½ cup shredded Gruyère cheese
1½ teaspoons fresh chopped rosemary leaves

Preheat the oven to 400°F.

Put the potatoes in a large saucepan with enough water to cover. Bring to a boil and cook for 5 minutes. Drain in a colander. When potatoes have cooled and can be handled, slice thin.

Unfold the dough and roll into a 10-by-9-inch rectangle. Cut into about twenty bite-size squares.

Score the edges with a fork, and prick the dough all over with fork tines.

Lay the squares on a baking sheet and refrigerate for 10 minutes. Remove from refrigerator.

In a small bowl, mix together the cheese and the rosemary leaves. Add a big pinch of the cheese mixture to each potato slice, and place each slice on a phyllo square.

Bake for 15 minutes or until golden brown. Serve.

Crispy Chickpeas

Put these in small bowls and scatter around as appetizers and for snacking. These chickpeas will delight you with a crunchy satisfaction usually reserved for fried snack foods like potato chips. They can be enjoyed during all phases of your diet.

2 cans (15.5 ounces) chickpeas (garbanzo beans), drained and rinsed
1 teaspoon ground cumin
½ teaspoon salt
2 garlic cloves, minced

Preheat the oven to 300°F.

Put the chickpeas in a towel and rub off the skins. Discard the skins.

In a large bowl, thoroughly mix skinned chickpeas, cumin, salt, and garlic.

Spread the chickpeas on a baking sheet and bake for 1 hour and 30 to 40 minutes, stirring every 20 minutes to ensure browning all over. Serve.

Almost Tzatziki

Based on the Greek dish of the same name, this "tzatziki" uses dill instead of mint, as the oils in mint trigger acid reflux. You can certainly try the mint and see if your chemistry rebels, but dill or cilantro will surely soothe your food pipe and bring down inflammation.

1 cup grated English cucumber
1 cup plain nonfat Greek yogurt
1 tablespoon chopped dill or cilantro
2 garlic cloves, minced

Put all ingredients together in the bowl of a food processor and pulse until combined. Pour into a small bowl and refrigerate for at least 30 minutes.

Serve with triangles of toasted whole-wheat pita wedges.

Appetizers and Side Dishes

Glazed Carrots

Carrot coins and butter create shiny, perfectly glazed vegetables that make for a tempting side dish—not to mention cooked carrots have a great pH for the GERD patient at 6.03.

6 large carrots, peeled and cut into 1-inch-thick coins
2 to 3 tablespoons butter
¼ teaspoon salt
Splash of fresh lemon juice

In a large saucepan, boil the carrot coins until firm to the touch yet softened, then drain.

In a large frying pan over medium heat, melt the butter. Add the carrots and stir. Add the salt and lemon juice and stir again. Continue to heat and stir until the carrots are shiny and completely coated in butter and seasoning. Serve.

Broccoli and Cheese

SERVES 4

Broccoli is a go-to food for human health: you simply cannot eat enough of it. Broccoli has a pH above 6, making it perfect throughout an eating program for acid reflux. There's not enough acid in the mustard to affect this pH.

1 head broccoli, cut into bite-size florets
4 ounces cheddar cheese, grated
2 teaspoons prepared Dijon mustard

Steam the broccoli until firm-tender.

In a medium bowl, combine the cheese and mustard, and then add the steamed broccoli and mix.

Microwave on high for 1 to 2 minutes or, alternatively, heat under the broiler for 3 to 4 minutes or until the cheese is melted. Serve.

Perfect Mashed Potatoes

Potatoes are above a 5 on the pH scale, and when you lace them with butter and milk the pH drops even lower. The secret to great mashed potatoes is to use Yukon gold potatoes—that's how to get a creamy consistency. This dish is an appropriate choice throughout all phases of the Acid Reflux Diet.

6 Yukon gold potatoes, peeled
2 to 3 tablespoons unsalted butter
½ teaspoon salt
2 to 3 tablespoons low-fat milk

In a large pot, cook the potatoes in boiling water until firm-done. Drain.

In a large bowl, combine the potatoes, butter, salt, and milk.

Mash with a potato masher, ricer, or electric mixer. Serve immediately.

Prevent Acid Reflux

Delicious Cabbage

SERVES 4

Cabbage gets a bad rap because of the way it smells while cooking. To combat this, add a little salt and lemon juice to the water—it pours off but contains the smell. Cabbage is a perfect vegetable to combat acid reflux during all phases of treatment.

1 head cabbage, cored and cut into thin slices
2 tablespoons unsalted butter
Splash of lemon juice
½ teaspoon salt

Fill a large saucepan with water and bring it to a boil. Add the cabbage and boil until firm-tender. Drain.

Return the dry saucepan to the stove. Add the butter and melt over medium heat.

Increase to medium-high and add the cabbage. Add lemon juice and salt. Sauté for 4 to 5 minutes, stirring frequently, and serve.

Roasted Brussels Sprouts with Butter and Cheese

Like broccoli, Brussels sprouts have their fans. If you are one of them, try this recipe; its pH is perfect for the rest of your life.

3 tablespoons unsalted butter, melted
3 cups halved Brussels sprouts, outer rough, yellow leaves removed
¼ teaspoon salt
2 tablespoons grated Parmesan cheese

Preheat the oven to 400°F.

In a small saucepan, melt the butter over medium heat. In a large bowl toss the sprouts with the melted butter. Add the salt and toss again.

Spread the sprouts on a baking sheet and bake for 35 to 40 minutes, turning every 10 minutes or so. Remove from the oven and sprinkle cheese over top. Cool slightly and serve.

Creamed Corn

SERVES 4

Corn is alkaline and its kernels are a wonderful addition to salads and soups. Cream the corn and it's even better. Feel free to eat this whenever you like.

8 ears corn
1 tablespoon flour
1 tablespoon sugar
3 tablespoons unsalted butter
1 cup heavy cream
½ cup water

In a large bowl, cut the end off a piece of corn, and hold it vertically in the base of the bowl with the stalk-end down. Using a paring knife, cut the kernels from the cob. After you complete a cob, run the back of the knife down its side to squeeze the juice into the bowl. Repeat until all the cobs are clean.

Mix the flour and sugar together in a small bowl. In a skillet over medium heat, melt 2 tablespoons of the butter. Add the corn kernels and juices and sprinkle the flour mixture over it. Stir to combine.

Stir in the cream and water and stir constantly until the mixture has thickened, 3 to 4 minutes. Serve.

Appetizers and Side Dishes

CHAPTER NINE

Main Courses

Roasted Vegetables with
Gruyère Cheese

Pasta and Roasted Vegetables with
Gruyère Cheese

Roasted Vegetable with Gruyère
Cheese Lasagna

Roasted Vegetable with Gruyère
Cheese "Pizzas"

Perfect Fish

Perfect Fish with Herbed Lemon Sauce

Roasted Fish on a Bed of Vegetables

Roasted Fish with Corn, Ginger,
and Cilantro

Shrimp and Corn

Fast Shrimp Pilaf

Individual Scotch Meat Loaves

Sweet-Potato Hash with Eggs

Pasta with Oil, Garlic, and Herbs

Creamy Peas with Pasta

Lentils and Kale

Stuffed Flounder

Avocado-Egg Salad in a
Whole-Wheat Wrap

Black-Bean and Portobello
Mushroom Quesadillas

Quick Vegetable Curry

CHAPTER NINE

Main Courses

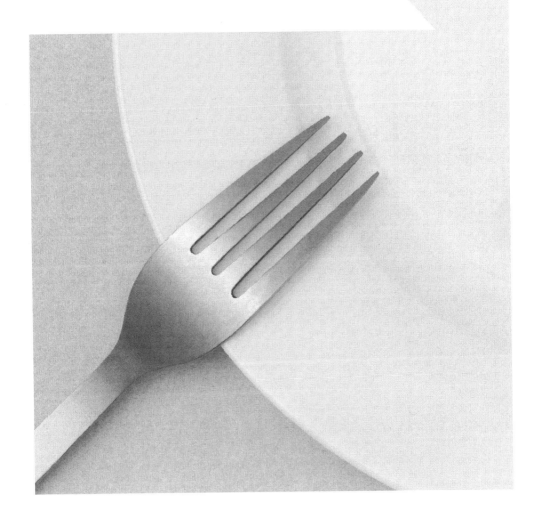

Roasted Vegetables with Gruyère Cheese

Roast root vegetables for an hour with extra-virgin olive oil, and serve on brown rice for a satisfying meal at any phase of your eating program. You'll find many uses for this dish: pile the veggies on whole-wheat bread or pitas for breakfast, lunch, or dinner.

2 large zucchini, cut into bite-size pieces
2 summer squash, cut into bite-size pieces
1 sweet potato, peeled and diced
2 to 3 tablespoons extra-virgin olive oil
Generous pinch of salt
⅓ cup shredded Gruyère cheese
2 cups cooked brown rice

Preheat the oven to 400°F.

In a medium-sized bowl, combine the prepared zucchini, squash, and sweet potato with the olive oil and salt, and toss to coat. Spread on a rimmed baking sheet and bake, turning over twice, until all the vegetables are roasted, about 1 hour.

When the vegetables are roasted, sprinkle cheese on top and bake for another 3 to 5 minutes, or until the cheese melts. Serve on top of brown rice.

Pasta and Roasted Vegetables with Gruyère Cheese

SERVES 4

Roasted Vegetables with Gruyère Cheese is perfect to toss with warm pasta and extra-virgin olive oil. Once you have roasted the vegetables, you'll have dinner ready for the workweek to come: this mix can be stored covered in the refrigerator and used repeatedly. Just reheat the vegetables and create meal after meal.

Roasted Vegetables with Gruyère Cheese (page 111)
1 pound spaghetti, cooked
1 to 2 tablespoons extra-virgin olive oil

In a large bowl, toss the hot vegetable mixture and the cooked pasta. Add olive oil if more moisture is needed and serve immediately.

Prevent Acid Reflux

Roasted Vegetable with Gruyère Cheese Lasagna

SERVES 4 TO 6

This lasagna turns humble roasted vegetables into a dish worthy of an elegant dinner or casual meal in front of the Sunday game. It's perfect for Phase I or II of your diet. If you like, try experimenting with cheeses, substituting fontina for the Gruyère.

1 (12- or 16-ounce) package lasagna noodles, depending
    on size of pan
1 tablespoon extra-virgin olive oil
3 tablespoons unsalted butter
2 garlic cloves, minced
¼ cup flour
3½ cups milk
4 tablespoons finely grated Parmigiano-Reggiano cheese
Roasted Vegetables with Gruyère Cheese (page 111)

Preheat the oven to 425°F.

Cook the noodles according the package instructions, drain, and toss with the olive oil to keep the noodles from sticking. Set aside.

To make the sauce: In a frying pan or medium saucepan, melt the butter over medium heat. Add the garlic and sauté until soft but not brown.

Add the flour, and stir constantly for 1 minute. Pour the milk into the pan slowly, whisking constantly. Continue to whisk as the milk thickens, about 2 minutes. Remove from the heat, and stir in 2 tablespoons of the cheese.

To assemble the lasagna: Spread a tablespoon or two of the sauce across the bottom of a 9-by-13-inch casserole dish. Layer noodles on top, then a cup of vegetables. Add another layer of noodles, then another cup of vegetables, and continue layering thus, stacking up to the top of the pan. The final layer should be noodle.

Pour the sauce over the stack of vegetables and noodles. Sprinkle the final 2 tablespoons of grated cheese over the top and bake for 25 minutes. Remove and let sit for 10 minutes before serving.

Roasted Vegetable with Gruyère Cheese "Pizzas"

SERVES 4

Warm, satisfying, and delicious, these pizzas can be assembled quickly when you have roasted vegetables on hand. Eat as breakfast, lunch, dinner, or have half an English muffin covered in vegetables for a snack. This is a go-to recipe for both phases of your diet.

4 whole-wheat English muffins, split in half and toasted
1 garlic clove, cut in half
Roasted Vegetables with Gruyère Cheese (page 111)

Preheat the broiler of an oven or set a toaster oven to broil.

While the muffins are still warm, rub the cut garlic over each cut surface for flavor. Mound a heaping tablespoon or more of vegetable mixture on each muffin half. Arrange on a baking sheet.

Heat the muffins under the broiler for 2 to 3 minutes or until the vegetables are hot and the cheese melted. Serve immediately.

Perfect Fish

This technique makes flawless golden-brown fish filets, a perfect food to combat acid reflux. These filets also make a great sandwich. Dress it with a combination of Greek yogurt, a pinch of salt, and dried oregano in place of tartar sauce.

2 tablespoons extra-virgin olive oil
2 (4- to 6-ounce) filets salmon, Arctic char, or monkfish
½ teaspoon salt
1 lemon, quartered

Preheat the oven to 450°F.

Rub olive oil on both sides of the filets, and sprinkle with a little salt.

Heat a large ovenproof frying pan on high until a drop of water sizzles on the pan and evaporates.

Place the filets in the pan, skin-side down. Cook until the skin is brown and crusty, then flip the filets. Slide the frying pan into the preheated oven.

Roast for 7 to 10 minutes or until the other side of the fish is golden, and the skin has a crunchy crust. Serve immediately with 2 lemon wedges.

Main Courses

Perfect Fish with Herbed Lemon Sauce

Here's a different way to roast the perfect fish. The lemon is diffused and shouldn't trigger your symptoms. Serve this over a bed of rice, preferably brown.

Juice of 1 lemon
3 garlic cloves, minced
1 cup coarsely chopped parsley
¼ cup chopped basil leaves
⅓ cup extra-virgin olive oil
Perfect Fish (page 115)

In a small bowl, combine the lemon juice, garlic, parsley, basil, and olive oil.

Mix thoroughly with a whisk, or put in a jar with a lid and shake until combined. Set aside.

Prepare Perfect Fish.

When you remove the fish from the oven, let it rest for a minute, then pour the sauce around it and let sit for 2 to 3 minutes more.

Serve with rice on a plate, laying a fish filet on top of the rice and pouring the sauce over all.

Roasted Fish on a Bed of Vegetables

This is another version of a perfect fish filet cooked atop vegetables with a healing pH. Serve with a side of brown rice.

1 cup roughly chopped baby carrots
1 cup roughly chopped summer squash
3 tablespoons extra-virgin olive oil
Pinch of salt
Perfect Fish (page 115)

Preheat the oven to 450°F.

In an ovenproof casserole dish, toss the carrots and squash with the olive oil and salt. Roast, turning once, for 30 minutes.

Prepare Perfect Fish.

When the fish is ready to roast, simply transfer it from the stove top directly to the vegetables in the oven, roasting all for 7 to 10 minutes.

Main Courses

Roasted Fish with Corn, Ginger, and Cilantro

SERVES 2

These four ingredients—fish, corn, fresh ginger, and cilantro—are some of the most soothing ingredients ever for the GERD sufferer.

Perfect Fish (page 115)
2 tablespoons unsalted butter
1 tablespoon extra-virgin olive oil
½ cup green onions, white and green parts thinly sliced
Pinch of salt
2 cups fresh corn kernels
1 tablespoon fresh minced ginger
1 tablespoon fresh minced garlic
3 tablespoons fresh chopped cilantro leaves
Juice of ½ lime

Prepare Perfect Fish.

As the fish roasts, prepare the corn topping by melting the butter and oil in a large saucepan over medium-high heat. Add the green onions and salt and cook for approximately 3 minutes. Remove.

In a large mixing bowl, combine corn kernels, ginger, and garlic, then stir in the cooled green onions and cilantro leaves. Squeeze lime juice over all, mix thoroughly, and set aside.

Remove the fish from the oven and place each filet in the middle of a plate. Heap the corn mixture on top and serve immediately.

Shrimp and Corn

SERVES 4

Use the recipe for Corn, Ginger, and Cilantro as your foundation and top it with your protein of choice. Instead of fish, here we use shrimp, another seafood that has the right pH for your needs. Alternatively, toss on small cubes of fried tofu.

Corn, Ginger, and Cilantro (page 118, omitting the fish)
1 pound shrimp, boiled, shelled, and deveined

Prepare Corn, Ginger and Cilantro, omitting the roasted fish.

In a large stockpot, cook the shrimp in salted boiling water until just pink (about 3 minutes). Drain in a colander. Run under cold water until cool enough to handle.

Place the corn mixture in the center of a plate and add one-fourth of the shrimp on top. Repeat until you have 4 plates of corn and shrimp. Serve.

Main Courses

Fast Shrimp Pilaf

SERVES 4

Many of the world's great cuisines pair shrimp and rice. Learn your trigger foods and you can adjust these recipes to fit your new lifestyle. Just leave out foods that irritate your chemistry by omitting troublesome ingredients and adding in new ones.

Don't worry—this isn't about "authentic" cooking, it's about you feeling better.

1 tablespoon canola oil
½ cup diced onion
1 cup diced green bell pepper
1 tablespoon minced garlic
2 teaspoons Old Bay seasoning
1 pound shrimp, shelled and deveined
1 (8-ounce) bottle clam juice
Squeeze of fresh lemon juice
1½ cups instant rice

In a large frying pan, heat the oil over medium-high until it shines. Add the onion and pepper, and cook for 2 minutes.

Add the garlic and seasoning, and cook for 1 minute.

Add the shrimp, clam juice, lemon juice, and rice. Mix and cover the pan. Remove from the heat and let sit for 5 minutes.

Uncover, return to the stove, and cook for 1 minute longer, heating through completely. Serve.

Individual Scotch Meat Loaves

Ground turkey hovers around a pH of 5 or above. The leaner the meat, the better for your condition in the first phase of the diet. Add in your favorite ground spices as your health improves, and make this a staple of Phase II.

1 tablespoon vegetable oil
½ cup chopped onion
1 egg
½ cup skim milk
1 cup long-cooking oatmeal, raw
1 pound ground turkey, preferably lean white meat
Pinch of salt
½ teaspoon ground sage
Splash of Worcestershire sauce
4 hard-boiled eggs, peeled

Preheat the oven to 375°F.

In a small frying pan, heat the oil over medium-high. Add the onion and sauté until soft and translucent, about 5 minutes. Remove.

In a large mixing bowl, beat the egg and then whisk in the milk. Add the oatmeal and let sit for 5 to 10 minutes as the oatmeal absorbs the liquid.

Add the turkey, salt, sage, and Worcestershire sauce, and mix all ingredients together with your hands until combined.

Separate the mixture into four equal parts. Take one part and form it around a hard-boiled egg, creating a small individual loaf. Lay on a baking sheet. Repeat until you have 4 loaves.

Slide into the oven and bake for 30 to 40 minutes. Serve.

Sweet-Potato Hash with Eggs

Obviously a recipe that's ideal for breakfast or brunch, Sweet-Potato Hash makes a deeply satisfying, casual supper. Serve with a piece of whole-wheat bread slathered with unsalted butter.

2 tablespoons unsalted butter
1 cup diced onion
1 teaspoon plus pinch of salt
2 large sweet potatoes, peeled and diced into 1-inch cubes
½ pound lean ground turkey, cooked until crisp
3 large garlic cloves, minced
2 tablespoons fresh rosemary leaves, minced
4 eggs

Preheat the oven to 425°F.

In a cast-iron skillet over medium-high heat, melt the butter. Add the onion and pinch of salt. Cook until brown, about 30 minutes, stirring frequently, then remove from heat.

Put the potatoes in a large bowl. Add the browned turkey and the onion mixture, and combine thoroughly. Add the garlic, rosemary, and the teaspoon of salt, and toss.

Spread the sweet potato mixture on a rimmed baking sheet and bake for 30 minutes.

Transfer back into the clean cast-iron skillet.

Make four wells in the sweet potato mixture, and crack an egg into each. Put the skillet in the oven and bake for 15 minutes, until the eggs are set and firm. Serve an egg to each person with a heaping spoonful or two of the hash.

Pasta with Oil, Garlic, and Herbs

SERVES 4

This simple recipe provides a soothing, low-acid pasta dish.

1 pound pasta, spaghetti or penne
½ cup olive oil
4 garlic cloves, thinly sliced
¼ cup chopped parsley
¼ cup chopped basil
½ cup grated Parmesan cheese

Cook pasta according to the package instructions. Drain.

While the pasta cooks, heat the oil in a saucepan or small skillet. When the oil is hot and shiny, add the garlic and cook for 2 to 3 minutes until soft, but not brown.

Add pasta, hot oil, and garlic to a large serving bowl and toss.

When completely combined, add the parsley and basil and toss again. Divide between four plates and serve with grated Parmesan.

Main Courses

Creamy Peas with Pasta

SERVES 4

A soothing dish that's full of alkaline ingredients, this pasta is easy to prepare and an excellent solution for a quick weeknight dinner. It's also good for all phases of your recovery.

1 pound pasta, such as bow-ties (farfalle), penne, or rigatoni
½ cup heavy cream
½ cup vegetable broth
Juice of ½ lemon
2 cups frozen peas
½ cup grated Parmesan cheese
¼ cup chopped parsley

Cook pasta according to the package instructions. Drain.

In a small saucepan, whisk together the cream and vegetable broth, and heat over medium-high. When the mixture is close to boiling, add the lemon juice, peas, and cheese. When the pan returns to a boil, lower the temperature to a simmer and cook for 6 to 8 minutes, until the peas are soft.

In a large bowl, toss the pasta with the creamy pea mixture. Add the parsley and continue to toss until mixed. Serve immediately.

Prevent Acid Reflux

Lentils and Kale

This is a soupy, juicy bowl of protein and nutrients, all strongly alkaline for the reflux stomach. Eat this chunky, rustic dish with a big hunk of crusty whole-wheat bread.

2 tablespoons extra-virgin olive oil
1 cup shredded carrot
¼ cup finely chopped onion
4 garlic cloves, minced
4 cups low-sodium, low-fat vegetable broth
1 (16-ounce) package lentils
1 bunch kale, washed, stems removed, and torn into pieces
¼ cup grated Pecorino-Romano cheese

In a stockpot over medium-high, heat the oil until it shines. Add the carrot, onion, and garlic. Sauté until all the vegetables are softened, about 3 to 4 minutes.

Add the broth to the pan and bring to a boil. Add the lentils and cook for 30 to 40 minutes, or until the lentils are cooked.

Add the kale and cook for 4 to 5 minutes more. Divide among four bowls, sprinkle cheese on top of each, and serve immediately.

Main Courses

Stuffed Flounder

SERVES 4

Delicate flounder filets are alkaline and can register almost a 7 on the pH scale. Roll this fish around in crabmeat (another alkaline seafood) and vegetables sautéed in butter for a memorable evening meal. Serve alongside rice or lightly oiled pasta combined with chopped fresh herbs such as parsley, dill, chives, or fresh oregano.

5 tablespoons unsalted butter
2 tablespoons minced celery
1 tablespoon minced garlic
2 tablespoons minced green bell pepper
¾ pound crabmeat, picked over and cartilage removed
1 egg, beaten
½ cup bread crumbs
1 pound flounder filets, rinsed and dried

Preheat the oven to 350°F.

In a small frying pan or saucepan over medium-high heat, melt 3 tablespoons of the butter.

Add the celery, garlic, and pepper, and cook until softened, stirring frequently, for about 3 minutes. Remove and let cool.

In a large bowl mix crabmeat with beaten egg and ¼ cup of the bread crumbs.

Lay the flounder filets on a clean surface. Mound the crabmeat mixture in the center of each filet, roll the filet around it, and secure with a toothpick, if necessary.

Place the rolled flounder filets, toothpick-side down, in an oiled casserole pan or baking sheet.

Repeat until all the filets are stuffed. Sprinkle the other ¼ cup of bread crumbs over the fish. Melt the 2 remaining tablespoons of butter and drizzle over the rolled fish filets.

Bake for 20 minutes and serve immediately.

Avocado-Egg Salad in a Whole-Wheat Wrap

SERVES 2

This roll-up sandwich is in the main dish section because it's an easy dinner for those nights when you are just too tired—or it's simply too hot outside—to cook. This is a recipe you can use for life.

4 hard-boiled eggs, peeled
1 large, soft, ripe avocado, pitted and flesh scooped out
1 tablespoon plain low-fat Greek yogurt
1 teaspoon curry powder
Pinch of salt
2 whole-wheat large tortillas or sandwich roll-ups
¼ cup lettuce such as butter, curly green, or romaine, shredded

Cut the eggs into quarters. In a medium mixing bowl, mash the eggs with the back of a fork until broken into smaller pieces. Add the avocado and continue to mash until completely combined. Add the yogurt, curry powder, and salt, and continue mashing.

Lay a wrap on a clean surface, and mound half the egg mixture on it so that it reaches about an inch from the edge. Add half the shredded lettuce, and roll the egg mixture inside the wrap. Repeat with the remaining wraps. Serve immediately.

Black-Bean and Portobello Mushroom Quesadillas

Mushrooms and black beans sink into melted cheese in these quesadillas, creating an excellent, quick dinner for any phase of the Acid Reflux Diet at any time.

4 tablespoons unsalted butter
2 garlic cloves, minced
4 large portobello mushroom caps, thinly sliced
1 cup low-sodium canned black beans, drained and rinsed
1 cup shredded Mexican cheese blend
4 (8-inch) whole-wheat or flour tortillas

In a small frying pan or saucepan over medium-high heat, melt 1 tablespoon of the butter.

Add the garlic, stir, and cook for 2 minutes, or until the garlic is soft and fragrant. Add the mushroom slices and cook, stirring frequently, until the mushrooms grow soft, shiny, and release their liquid, 5 or 6 minutes. Remove from heat and allow to cool slightly.

In a large mixing bowl, combine the beans, cheese, and mushroom mixture.

In a large frying pan over medium heat, melt the remaining butter.

Meanwhile, spread half the vegetable mixture over a tortilla, and cover with another tortilla. Transfer to the frying pan, and cook for 3 minutes. Flip and cook another 3 minutes, or until all the cheese is melted. Serve immediately.

Repeat the process with the other tortillas.

Quick Vegetable Curry

SERVES 4

Believe it or not, curry registers alkaline. This speedy, soupy curry filled with vegetables gives you fiber, nutrients, and warm comfort. Serve with crusty bread over couscous (quickest cooking of the grains) or brown rice. This dish is a first-rate choice for any time in your diet.

1 large head broccoli, cut into small florets
1 tablespoon curry powder
1 teaspoon cumin
1 (15-ounce) can chickpeas (garbanzo beans), drained and rinsed
1 (15-ounce) can frozen peas
2 large red potatoes, diced
1 cup canned pumpkin
1 cup water
1 (13.5-ounce) can coconut milk

In a large saucepan over high heat, bring salted water to a boil. Add the broccoli florets and blanch for 3 minutes. Drain.

In a large skillet over medium heat, cook the curry and cumin, stirring constantly, for 30 seconds or until fragrant. Add the chickpeas, frozen peas, potatoes, pumpkin, water, coconut milk, and broccoli florets. Mix thoroughly, reduce the heat to medium, and simmer for 15 minutes. Serve over couscous or brown rice.

Desserts

CHAPTER TEN
Desserts

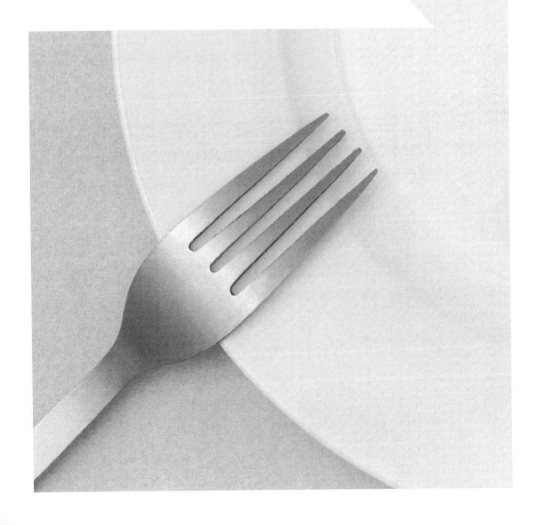

Mixed Summer Melons with Honey Cream

Melons are refreshing, light, and have the perfect pH to end a meal.

1 honeydew melon, flesh cut into bite-size pieces
1 cantaloupe, flesh cut into bite-size pieces
Juice of ½ lemon
½ cup plain low-fat Greek yogurt
2 tablespoons honey
¼ cup pecans, chopped

In a mixing bowl, combine the melon, cantaloupe, and lemon juice, tossing well. (This will keep the melon from oxidizing and turning brown, a function of acid.)

In another small bowl, mix the yogurt and honey.

Spoon the melon into a serving bowl, add a heaping tablespoon of yogurt, and top with chopped pecans. Serve.

Marshmallow Graham-Cracker Sandwiches

SERVES 4

Marshmallow is a soothing substance on an inflamed food pipe. This is a s'more without the chocolate, because chocolate is a huge trigger for many who fight acid reflux. Graham crackers have a pH of around 7 and are a great food for snacking in moderation. For an extra twist of flavor, add a dash of cinnamon or nutmeg on top of the marshmallow before you close the sandwich.

¾ cup sugar

1 tablespoon corn syrup

¼ cup milk

½ (16-ounce) package marshmallows, coarsely chopped

1 to 2 tablespoons water

1 wax-paper sleeve of graham crackers

In a small saucepan over medium heat, combine the sugar, corn syrup, and milk. Cook, stirring constantly, until sugar is melted and combined, about 5 minutes.

In a double boiler with an inch of water in the bottom pan, combine the marshmallows and water. Cook, stirring constantly, until melted. Add to the sugar mixture and combine thoroughly.

Split each graham cracker in half. Add a heaping tablespoon of marshmallow mixture and cover with the other half. Repeat until all the marshmallow has been used. Serve.

Avocado Pie

Unusual and delicious, Avocado Pie also makes a good afternoon snack. An interesting note on cream cheese: it becomes more alkaline when you beat it. This is a rich, soothing pie, so a thin slice is all you need.

2 large, soft, ripe avocados, flesh scooped out
1 (8-ounce) package low-fat or nonfat cream cheese
1 (14-ounce) can sweetened condensed milk
3 tablespoons fresh lime juice
1 ready-made graham cracker crust
1 cup heavy cream
1 tablespoon sugar

In a large bowl, combine the avocado, cream cheese, condensed milk, and lime juice. Beat with an electric mixer until creamy.

Pour the avocado mixture into the pie crust and refrigerate for at least 4 hours.

When you are ready to serve, beat the cream and sugar together with an electric mixer until the cream is firm and forms stiff peaks. Mound the cream in the middle of the pie and spread outward. Serve immediately.

Desserts

Sweet Potato Pie

Sweet potatoes are a perfect food, naturally sweet and just the right base for a pie. Take small wedges with you and eat as a snack on the road.

3 tablespoons flour
1¼ cups sugar
½ teaspoon ground nutmeg
Pinch of salt
1½ cups mashed sweet potato
2 eggs
¼ cup light corn syrup
½ cup unsalted butter
¾ cup evaporated milk
1 store-bought pie crust

Preheat the oven to 350°F.

In a small bowl, combine the flour, sugar, nutmeg, and salt. In a larger mixing bowl, beat the sweet potato, eggs, corn syrup, butter, and milk with a handheld mixer.

Slowly add the flour mix to the sweet-potato mixture, beating on low until all is combined. Pour into the pie crust and bake for 1 hour or until a toothpick inserted in the center of the pie comes out clean. Let cool for 10 minutes and serve in small wedges.

Prevent Acid Reflux

Tropical Fruit Parfaits

SERVES 2

Layer soothing tropical fruits such as mango and papaya in between Greek yogurt whipped with a touch of cinnamon—delicious!

1 cup papaya, cut into bite-size chunks
1 cup mango, cut into bite-size chunks
Juice of ½ lemon
1 cup plain low-fat Greek yogurt
1½ teaspoons cinnamon

In a mixing bowl, combine the fruit and lemon juice, and mix thoroughly.

In a small bowl, whisk together the yogurt and cinnamon.

In two large wine or brandy glasses, layer the fruit with yogurt, and repeat until the glass is full. Serve immediately.

Quick Banana-Nut Bread

This quick and easy banana bread has more banana and less sugar than most. Toast slices and slather with a tablespoon of unsalted butter for a snack.

Cooking spray, such as PAM
1½ cups self-rising flour
½ cup sugar
1 teaspoon extra-virgin olive oil
3 tablespoons milk
2 eggs, lightly beaten
1¼ cups ripe mashed bananas
½ cup pecans, chopped

Preheat the oven to 350°F.

Spray a standard loaf pan with cooking spray.

In a medium bowl, whisk together the flour and sugar. Add the oil, milk, and eggs, and mix well. Add the bananas and pecans and stir, then pour into the prepared loaf pan.

Bake for 55 to 60 minutes or until a toothpick comes out clean. Let sit for 10 minutes, tip the loaf pan over a plate to release, and serve.

Fluffy, Lemony Sweet Cheese Pudding

SERVES 4

If you whip low-fat cottage cheese and fold it into slightly sweetened whipped cream, you create an airy dessert, much like a light pudding.

3 cups low-fat cottage cheese
Juice of ½ lemon
1 cup whipping cream
2 tablespoons sugar

In a medium bowl, beat the cottage cheese and lemon juice with a handheld mixer. Set aside.

In a larger bowl, whip the cream with the sugar. Fold the stiffened cream into the cottage-cheese mixture. Refrigerate for at least 2 hours and serve.

Fresh Figs, Almonds, and Manchego Cheese

SERVES 4

Figs, almonds, and Manchego are deeply embedded in Spanish cuisine. Try Marcona almonds if you crave authenticity.

8 figs, split
½ cup Marcona almonds, coarsely chopped
2 to 3 tablespoons grated Manchego cheese
2 tablespoons honey
2 tablespoons balsamic vinegar

Arrange the figs on a platter. Sprinkle the chopped almonds on the figs, then sprinkle with cheese. Drizzle honey and vinegar over all, and serve immediately.

Vanilla Pudding

What could be more soothing to a savage stomach? You can whip up this simple dessert right before dinner, then refrigerate and enjoy.

½ cup granulated sugar
2 tablespoons corn syrup
¼ teaspoon salt
3 cups whole milk
3 large egg yolks, beaten
2 teaspoons vanilla extract

In a small saucepan, mix the sugar, corn syrup, and salt. Slowly whisk in ¼ cup of the milk, then the egg yolks and vanilla, then the remaining milk.

Put the saucepan on the stove over medium heat, whisking constantly for 3 to 5 minutes until the mixture thickens.

Remove from heat and pour into individual ramekins, small glasses, or serving bowls. Put plastic wrap over the surface of each dish, and refrigerate for 2 hours before serving.

Snickerdoodles

Snickerdoodles are vanilla cookies with cinnamon and sugar on top, just the thing for the acid-prone food pipe and stomach. Try using two Snickerdoodles as the "bread" in a sandwich of frozen vanilla yogurt or slightly sweetened whipped cream.

½ cup unsalted butter, room temperature
½ cup vegetable shortening
1¼ cups plus 2 tablespoons sugar
2 eggs
2 cups flour
2 teaspoons cream of tartar
1 teaspoon baking soda
½ teaspoon salt
1 tablespoon cinnamon

Preheat the oven to 400°F.

In a bowl with a handheld mixer, beat together the butter, shortening, 1¼ cups of the sugar, and eggs until smooth, about 1 to 2 minutes.

In another bowl, sift together the flour, cream of tartar, baking soda, and salt. Stir into the butter mixture and combine thoroughly.

In a small bowl, mix together the remaining 2 tablespoons sugar with the cinnamon.

Take a heaping tablespoon of the butter and flour mixture, form into a ball, and dip the top of the ball in the sugar and cinnamon. Press it into the cookie with the back of a fork, leaving tine marks and flattening the cookie slightly. Place cookies 2 inches apart on an ungreased baking sheet and bake for 8 to 10 minutes. Remove and cool. Repeat process with remaining dough.

Prevent Acid Reflux

Resources

The website www.fda.gov offers the FDA's listing of the pH of common foods. Use it day in and day out for cooking and eating decisions.

Additional information on acid reflux and GERD can be found at:

advances.nutrition.org

nlm.nih.gov/medlineplus

www.health.harvard.edu

www.webmd.com

www.mayoclinic.com

Index

145

Index

148

Index

Made in the USA
Lexington, KY
09 March 2015